RECOVERING MY LIFE

How I decided bariatric surgery was right for me, the ups and downs of transformational weight loss, and why I would do it all over again.

CAROL ADKISSON

Paperback ISBN 978-1-7324242-0-3

Hardback ISBN 978-1-7324242-1-0

Library of Congress Control Number: 2017937453

Published by: Zoe Life Publications, Inc. DBA Anthology Inspired Press Post Office Box 310096 Fontana, CA 92331 www.aipress.info

First editor: Aisha S. Davis Second editor: Carol Rose Adkisson Cover illustration: Todd Adkisson Cover and text layout: TABIA Graphics

Photographer Danielle Jones: Facebook.com/ Seasonedwithsaltphotography

FB Status = Facebook Status

Publishing Services provided by Paper Raven Books

Printed in the United States of America

Author's Statement of Limitations: This is a real depiction of my own personal story. I am a Licensed Marriage and Family Therapist and I want it to be clear that my scope of practice is not medical in nature. I am not a doctor, or a nutritionist. I am not qualified to give medical advice. Please seek your own doctor's recommendations on all matters that affect your personal health.

TABLE OF CONTENTS

DEDICATION

I dedicate this book to my family, who went through every step of this process with me, from start to finish. They experienced the surgery with me, my ups and downs, and managed through their own feelings during this time. On top of all of that, they also were a part of every step of me writing this book; believing in the possibility that this can make a difference in someone's life. They gave up their time away from me in order for me to follow through with this labor of love. I love you all and I consider each one of you a participant in this book writing process.

ACKNOWLEDGEMENTS

Special thanks to the following:

My daughter Miranda, as the oldest child, and a daughter, you experienced this process in a different way from your siblings. From taking care of me post-op and shopping with this new strange looking mom, to the relationship that we have today that continues to help me be the role-model that you believe I am.

My son, Brian, who had to deal with a moody mom that was difficult to deal with and maybe still remains so at times. I appreciate your encouragement throughout these last few years. You never let me let go of the idea of this book becoming a reality. Thank you for that.

My son, Dylan, who also being the youngest, probably didn't understand all that I was going through during my surgery and afterward. However, you stepped up and helped me in the end, by researching information for this book and citing all of my references. I appreciate all the help that you gave me.

Todd, my husband, like Brian, wouldn't let me let go of this book being written. He never stopped encouraging me to complete this project so that I could make a difference in the lives of others. He was the first person that I read my entire book to. I took the risk that he wouldn't like it. He gave me so many things to think about throughout the first reading that helped me to create a much better book in the end. Thank you for everything. I will be forever grateful.

Charisse, my hairdresser, who gave me the makeover that I needed, and who has continued to be a good friend these past five years since I first became her hair model.

Cathy and her family, who put up with me, maybe too soon after my surgery, and helped me through the beginning stages of healing. Thank you.

Renee, for helping me to understand that having this surgery was not a definition of failure. She took care of my children while I recuperated, drove me to the hospital and sat with me until right before my surgery. Thank you for being my friend and helping me get through that first year.

Allen, for taking that picture of me at (the) La Brea Tar Pits. You probably didn't know it at the time, but this picture has become very important as my badge of courage.

Linda, who helped me to make it through my first speaking engagement, post-op, for making it painless when I was scared to death. Also for pushing me in a wheelchair and letting me be your first.

Steve, the psychologist who decided I was a good candidate for the surgery and helped me along the way in that first year post-op. You taught me a lot and I am grateful for that.

Mark, my life coach, who created a space of accountability that was the final catalyst for me completing this book.

To the helpful staff of both my primary doctor's office and my bariatric doctor's office, that helped me to become the woman I am today.

To the friends that have helped me along the way. There are too many of you to name. I couldn't have done this without your encouragement and support. I am blessed.

To Amanda, my friend and colleague. Thank you for your endless support and for reminding me that laughter is much better than taking life too seriously.

Finally to my publisher, Starla, thank you for believing in me and encouraging me all along the way, and for supporting me with the other books that we have worked on together. You are the best.

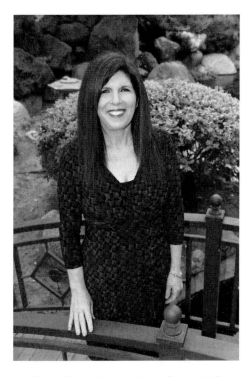

"Live Your Own Magnificent Life"
— Carol Rose Adkisson

"Remember to speak your own personal authentic voice. Your voice is unique, original, and needs to be heard."
—Carol Rose Adkisson

FOREWORD

Amanda Shannon M.A., LMFT

Being overweight steals from you. It will take anything and everything from you, down to your very life. If it hasn't taken your life, it will take your self-esteem, your dreams, your hopes, and even your relationships. You are in a fight for your life! Your future! Your family! You are fighting for YOU!!! Get angry at what this has cost you; use this to motivate you. Tell it, "NO MORE! You can no longer have my life, my future, my family, my hopes. You can no longer take from ME! I stand here reclaiming MY LIFE! I am taking it back!" Start believing you are worth it! You are important! You are needed! You are loved! Start dreaming Big Dreams for your future.

This is the very place Carol Adkisson found herself in the summer of 2009. She was not living life before the surgery, not the life God had intended for her. She tried to live life and hide her pain. At times, she did a good job at this – at times hiding her pain. But, even when hidden from the outside she was struggling on the inside.

I have been friends with Carol since 2000. We have done ministry, undergraduate and graduate programs together and even guided each other along our professional and personal paths. We went for walks together trying to fight this battle of obesity before her surgery. We would encourage each other to get moving and make wise choices. I have a lot of respect for her to get the courage to continue to fight the war of obesity. She fought for her life and it was not easy. She fought for her kids so they would have a mom. She fought for her future. She has put herself out there in hopes to inspire others to fight for their lives. For them to know the journey is not easy, but it is worth it. The journey is an important part of your developing the NEW YOU. She embraces her full journey and reshapes who she is as she tries to weed out unhealthy boundaries and parts of her life.

It is like she took off her cloak of shame and started to shine and show others who she is. This did not happen overnight, most journeys do not. But with one foot in front of the other she rebuilt her life, redefined herself, and embraced the challenges. Carol talks about how the world is opening up to her, living life to her full potential and how change is scary. You will see her mistakes, her successes, and tracking her weight loss journey and her health status.

I am a Licensed Marriage and Family Therapist, Child Mental Health Specialist, and Developmental Delay Mental Health Specialist. I have worked professionally as a Marriage and Family Therapist since 2008. I have also worked with many people struggling with addictions and trying to figure out how to do life healthy.

I hope you are encouraged by this book and that it helps you along your journey to find health and embracing the NEW YOU!

PREFACE

Let me introduce you to my personal journey. You will no doubt experience many emotions while reading this book. I will share the rollercoaster ride that I experienced both pre and post-surgery. My hope is that this book will encourage you in such a way that if you are going through this process, you can do it --- just as so many of us have. The aim of this book is to also help normalize every step that you are going through, or will go through.

With that caveat, please check with your doctor, as I am a therapist, not a medical practitioner. Through the 6½ years since my surgery, I have spoken to many people who have experienced this process, and every story is different. Try not to judge that you are doing it the wrong way. Instead, realize that your way is the right way for you. In the end, my hope is that you will come to terms with the fact that this surgery was a benefit to you and that you are happy you made the choice to say yes.

INTRODUCTION

Six and a half years ago, I had a gastric bypass. At that time, I was barely able to function as a productive person. Since then, I have been working on living the magnificent life. The dreams that I have always had have now become my new reality. My goal of being an authentic and productive person has been met and then some.

This book is written to bariatric patients that have been or will be in the weight loss process. I am a Licensed Marriage and Family Therapist. As a clinician that has been through the surgery personally, I wanted to share both my own personal journey and offer my hand up to encourage those in their own method of losing weight.

My credentials include a bachelor's degree from Hope International University in Human Development. I also received a Master's degree from Hope International University in Marriage and Family Therapy. I have a thriving group practice and a non-profit entitled, The Trauma and Healing Foundation. This foundation was created to assist people in our community to heal with the brokenness in their lives.

This book addresses many different areas. First, it tells one person's story and how her life changed. The story begins pre-surgery and continues primarily throughout the first year and a bit beyond. Second, it describes new ways in which to navigate your life to reach your goals and it helps to normalize what you may be going through. In other words, it lets you know that you are not alone; others are going through these same sorts of emotions, ideas, thoughts, etc. Third, it also shares what not to do, at least from the author's viewpoint. There is a chapter written directly to your friends and family, because they matter too. There is a chapter that describes the common types of bariatric surgery taken directly from the Mayo Clinic's website. In addition, there are a number of resources that may help you to educate yourself further, if you would like to do so. Finally, there are 44 videos that are made available for you, the reader, to see the raw unedited process that I went through during that first year.

This book was written as motivation to help encourage you to keep moving forward in obtaining your own magnificent life. Don't give up! One day at a time you can get there—you deserve to get there. Don't stop until you, too, can say that you are living out the person you were always meant to be.

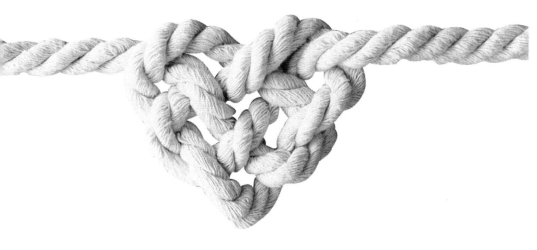

CHAPTER ONE

Pre-Surgery

My personal story is going to lead you on a journey through this new season in my life. Now, as I sit here six and a half years after my surgery, I can't believe the new person that I am now. However, this has been quite the process. I want to walk you through this journey and let you see who I was, what I went through, and who I have become, which will continue to evolve. My book is entitled *Recovering My Life, A Personal Bariatric Story*. Why did I call it that? Because I think it's important that anyone thinking about having the surgery and/ or someone who has had any type of bariatric surgery, to know the truth, the whole truth, at least from my perspective. All the good and the bad of the process and that through it all, I would do it again a million times over. However, I am a stubborn, did I say stubborn person, and thus I made a lot of mistakes along the way, which caused me to get where I was. That was needing the surgery and through the course, ending up in the hospital three months after the surgery. I am hoping that you won't make the mistakes that I did. I also hope that through the writing of this story with a touch of humor here and there, you can gain some information, so that you too can be successful.

Because of today's age of social networking, I have decided to write this book, as I was posting on social media in real life. I sprinkle throughout these chapters many of the FB Statuses that I posted on my personal Facebook page while I was losing weight. I also decided to include journal writings and video blogs that I did throughout most of my weight loss journey. Why you may ask? For several reasons; I figured it would help me to process through many of the feelings that I was having, too numerous to count at the time. Also, possibly to help someone else to feel encouraged to keep moving forward if they are going through the same things. For the first few months, I put myself in front of the camera and/or video at least once a week, and often many times more. In total, I have 44 videos of my progression. Which, by the way, for me took tremendous courage and was probably one of the hardest parts of this journey. Every time I saw myself in the camera, all I saw was how large my face was, and how many chins I had. I am making available with this book over two hours of videos of my first year post-surgery. The videos are a very real depiction of many of the thoughts that went through my head each day. As I look back through some of those thoughts, I almost don't know that person anymore. However, that was what I had to go through to become the new me, so that I could recover my life.

I do have a degree in Marriage and Family Therapy. In fact, as I am editing this, I am a Licensed Marriage and Family Therapist with a thriving practice. I have spoken at many events and I also have the Trauma and Healing Foundation, a non-profit organization. This foundation has been created to help make a difference in the community in many ways that includes; counseling, teaching classes, running process groups that cover various subject matters, conferences, and seminars. Because of my background, I had somewhat of an understanding of the emotional turmoil that I was going through. However, in this depiction, I am simply a patient relating her own personal experiences.

You know all of us get to this place (being morbidly obese) for different reasons. Many of us get to here through emotional eating and the need to avoid feelings through comfort eating. I was definitely one of those people. I ate because I didn't want men to want me. I didn't always consciously know that. However, it was true for me. I ate because I was broken inside due to childhood trauma. I ate because I was addicted to the feeling of not feeling. I ate because I liked the taste of food, too. Also I believe I had a genetic predisposition to weight issues. My dad struggled with weight loss, too. Although he didn't raise me, I have seen pictures of him up and down on the scale at various stages in his life. My mother was the opposite; she was the world's smallest woman and struggled with eating disorders that caused her to remain very small. These were some of the many reasons that I was overweight.

I spent most of my life trying to lose weight. This is not the place to go into the details; needless to say I had a rough life as a child. I have definitely been through things that a child should never have to go through. These things helped to formulate who I was as a child and contributed big time to the weight that I would begin to gain at a young age. And so I began the process of how my life was going to be. I remember dieting over and over again when I was in high school. I would lose the weight and then gain back even more. It always happened that way. In the beginning, I only needed to lose twenty or forty pounds. Eventually, I needed to lose more that one hundred pounds. I believe if I had continued in the way I was going, I would have continued to gain weight and the up and down roller coaster would have never stopped. I dieted using many different ideas. In high school, I ate nothing else but chicken and salads. I also exercised like an exercise addict. Doing 200 sit-ups was just the beginning for me. I could do hundreds and hundreds of them; whatever it took to lose the weight. As I began to get older, it wasn't as easy. I tried the grapefruit diet (I think), and the carb diet and the starvation diet, and the…, and the…, who-the-heck-knows-what-else diet. They all worked for a period of time, it just depended, until the weight began to sneak back onto my body or I reached a plateau. In time, I regained all the weight I had lost, plus more. I felt like my metabolism was the problem. Each year it required more and more to lose the weight. More exercise, more and longer dieting to get back to a normal weight. Until eventually it seemed like I couldn't do it anymore.

No diet or exercise plan seemed to work. By the time I was pregnant with my second child, I was over 200 pounds when I gave birth. That was the point where my medical problems began to increase. I finally was diagnosed with sleep apnea; it took many sleep studies to figure that one out. So then I required a c-pap machine, which only minimally helped the sleep deprivation that I had from non-restorative sleeping. I developed high cholesterol, I think when I was in my 30s and finally began to develop high blood pressure. I had hypoglycemia (low blood sugar) for as long as I can remember. When I was pregnant with my third child, it eventually became pre-diabetes and gestational diabetes.

In the end, I remember being unable to get out of bed. I was just too tired from my sleep apnea to function. I was feeling like the worst mom on the planet. I could barely accomplish the minimal for my kids during those years. I remember one especially painful and embarrassing time when I went to Knott's Berry Farm with my daughter; she was about nine I think. She was performing there as part of her choir in elementary school. I joined her there to watch her sing and we spent the day at the park. At one point we went into the kiddie section of the park and I went on a ride with her. Because it was a kid's ride, it was small. When the bar went across my waist (in order to keep us firmly in the ride), I felt this pop. That is the only way I can that I can think of how to describe what I felt.

Anyway, after I got off the ride, I went right to the bathroom because of the pain I felt in my bladder. I don't know exactly what happened, but somehow the way my organs were squeezed into that ride so tight, I caused myself a bladder infection. I wasn't the same for over a week after that. The pain was horrible, all because

I wanted to sit with my daughter in a ride and prove that I was like normal people. It's embarrassing to even recount that story.

During my years of grad school, I would crawl into my car and sleep between classes just to function and make it through my course load, which could last from 10 a.m. to 10 p.m. I am going to tell you a secret. I always tried to avert my eyes because I didn't want to see my reflection. I was too overweight and it embarrassed me to look at myself. At times, I couldn't resist it. I looked and realized that I looked just as bad as what I was afraid to see. Do you ever do that or feel that way? I was wearing size 16 pants at this point and realized they were beginning to become way too small. I was going to have to move up to a larger size before long.

I remember watching Carnie Wilson going through her surgery in front of the cameras some time ago. I knew I wasn't going to have that surgery, only slackers would do that. Then a friend of mine had the gastric bypass surgery and explained to me, based on her own understanding, that some people are weight loss resistant. In other words, they lose the weight but it always comes back on and then some. This planted a seed in me; I always felt that I had the worst metabolism in the world. I had lost 70 pounds more times than I could count and I had finally reached the point that I was rarely out of bed, mostly from sheer exhaustion from the sleep apnea. I began to formulate the idea that I would be willing to do the lap band. That was it, it would be easier and I gave into that idea. As God began to speak to my heart (yes, I am a Christian and the word God will be sprinkled throughout this book), I felt God tell me, "No, you are going to have the gastric bypass surgery." Stubborn as I am, I (in my mind) told Him no way, it wasn't going to happen. I don't need to do that. So the next time I went to the doctor, I cautiously brought up the weight loss surgery idea. I expected he would argue with me and say it was the easy way out or that he was against it. Instead he looked at me and said he had just gone to a conference on the subject and felt I would be an ideal candidate for the surgery. That certainly threw me for a loop, I didn't expect that response. Seriously, why couldn't he have just said the opposite and that would have been the end of it?

Because the doctor said yes, I began a new season in my life, fighting my way back to health. I had to fight for many reasons. To begin with, in order to get approved through my health insurance, it was necessary for my doctor and me to fight through the insurance approval system and not give up. One of my initial obstacles with getting the surgery was that I didn't want to go to the doctor in the first place. My main issue was that they weighed me each time I went in. I certainly didn't want to know what I weighed. Then, I got a bright idea; I can refuse to be weighed. You might ask why I didn't just tell them I didn't want to know my weight. Believe me, I told them that plenty of times. I averted my eyes from the scale and told them, "Don't tell me what I weigh." A second later, the nurse inadvertently slips out, "Oh Carol you weigh ..." Or the nurse follows through and doesn't tell me my weight, but then somehow the doctor works it into our consultation. I used to wonder if the medical staff just liked messing with me, revealing exactly what I didn't want to know. The truth probably is that there was a simple check in system at the doctor's office; a weight check is part of that system. How could the nurse or clerk possibly know that you are sensitive about hearing how much you weigh? I later learned, not weighing myself was a big hiccup in being approved by my insurance. "When it came time to consider the surgery, you have to show at least six months of trying to diet. It's important to show that even though you diet, your weight is not going down and staying down throughout the new eating plan. Unfortunately, my doctor could not document my weight from his files, since the information just wasn't in there. The chart likely said something like "patient refused to be weighed." That was my own fault. I refused to weigh myself for so long that there was no consistent record of my weight to report.

As I already have said, I had tried every diet known to man (slight exaggeration) and I already had met that criterion. In order to be considered for the surgery, I had to jump through the right hoops, be weighed enough times and the doctor had to document their assessment of my medical problems. I also needed to write a letter to my insurance company explaining the weight loss journey. I have a copy of this letter in Appendix A if you are interested in reading this. This is the process I went through. Like I said, every insurance company is different and every doctor is different. I can only tell my personal story and what I went through.

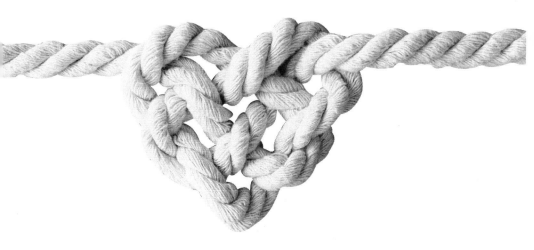

CHAPTER TWO

Preparing for the Day

I am sooooooo excited about this new season in my life. What does God have planned? All I know is that it is something great!
FB Status 8:52 p.m. April 26, 2010.

Once I got past the feeling that I would be a sellout if I had the surgery, I embraced it with everything in my being. I couldn't wait to know what I was going to feel like, look like, and act like after the surgery. I had been in the process of getting my surgery approved for quite some time. I felt like something amazing was going to happen in my life and I didn't have any idea what it was going to look like. I was excited and I couldn't wait for the surgery to happen. Before my surgery date, I began to look up people on the internet that had had the surgery. It was pretty cool; you could watch someone each week before and after his or her surgery date and see his or her weight loss. God, I wanted that so bad. I wanted to be one of those people that life begins to get better for. Their sicknesses went away, they felt healthier, and they seemed to be happier. And boy, they sure looked better. It seemed that life could change so much just from a simple operation. Maybe the surgery is not exactly that simple, but I wanted that. I wanted to be able to get out of bed in the morning and function all day and not feel like I hadn't slept in years.

As I watched those videos, I couldn't imagine the small portions they were eating. After all, I could eat an extra large pizza by myself in one sitting along with a salad and a drink. I sometimes visualized that I was actually stuffing my feelings down; not feeling them by eating so much. But then the shame always hit and I would feel worse about myself afterward. Emotional eating can be a viscous cycle.

Overeating can be an addiction. An addiction is something we use as a coping skill to not feel emotions. Along with addictions comes the guilt and shame of anyone finding out about our secret. As they say in 12-step programs, you are only as sick as your secrets. Do you have secrets? They can be so toxic to us. The problem with an eating addiction is that we all have to eat. There is no way getting around that. Now if I had an alcohol problem, I could simply chose to not drink ever again. How do you do that with food? I wondered if I could really become like the people on those videos who were able to change everything about their lives. I had hoped that I would find out that was true.

I remember thinking *why do people call me beautiful?* Many different people called me that. I wondered, *"Do they say that because they feel sorry for me, because they wanted me to feel beautiful even through I wasn't?"* I know that sounds like a crazy thought, but I didn't take them seriously. I always felt there was an ulterior motive to them calling me beautiful. I discounted any positive comments and embraced anything negative. I felt like some of their positive comments were pity in disguise and I was also called "smiley" a lot. I thought they said that because I was so optimistic. However, since the surgery, I have been told many times how much more upbeat I am. So, if I was upbeat before, what am I now? What was I really then? These are many of the thoughts that crossed my mind.

Today is the day that my surgery was approved. I was beginning to think that this day would never happen. I don't know when my surgery date is yet, but I do know that everything is going to change.

FB Status 12:27 a.m. May 25, 2010.

The doctor called to inform me that the insurance company asked for proof that I met the criteria to qualify for the surgery. In other words, was I overweight enough? I went into the office to be weighed to prove what my current weight was. What a surprise!. I still weighed enough for the surgery and then some. I met all the criteria to be approved for the surgery. This approval process felt so degrading and shaming. I couldn't wait until I didn't feel terrible getting on the scale.

Date Set for Surgery, Next Friday, June 4th. I will be in the hospital for 3-4 days. Any help would be appreciated. I'm scared, but excited; this is the beginning of a new season for me.

FB Status 3:48 p.m. May 25, 2010.

Omg, I got a call from the doctor, the date has been set for my surgery. It will be next Friday, June 4th. It is getting so close now and it is really real that this is going to happen. I don't even know what to feel.

Nine days until surgery. Will be in the hospital for 3-4 days. Any help would be appreciated.

FB Status 4:16 p.m. May 26, 2010.

Journal Entry #1:
I can't believe it is only nine days away. How did I get here? How is the surgery going to be? Will I be able to handle the pain? Lots of questions, not a lot of answers right now. I started realizing that I am going to need to exercise after the surgery. Although I love exercising, I am feeling a bit of pressure; probably from myself. What if I need plastic surgery after the weight loss? How

can I afford that? Will they approve me for that? I have so many racing thoughts going through my head.

Eight days until surgery. Will be in the hospital 3-4 days. Any help would be appreciated.
                              FB Status 10:30 a.m. May 27, 2010.

These FB Statuses were a cry for help. As I look back, I realized that I didn't have a clear voice and the ability to reach out and ask people directly for help. I was a single mom with three kids and I didn't know how I was going to provide for the needs of my three children, as well as take care of myself after the surgery. I couldn't take any risks beyond a FB Status, hoping others would read into my posting what I needed. Couldn't they just guess that I needed help?

I had spent a lifetime being afraid to ask for what I wanted. In fact, I can barely remember ever directly asking anyone for anything. This was something I needed to overcome and I didn't even know it back then. Nobody contacted me to help me. As a single mom, I became more and more concerned about my kids. Who would take care of me if I needed help? Who would take care of them, as they were young kids? My daughter was 15 years old. My boys were 13 and nearly 11 years old. I was so worried that I wouldn't be able to take care of my children and myself, too. I knew I had lots of friends. I just had to trust God in this.

Seven days until surgery. Will be in the hospital 3-4 days. Any help will be appreciated. Or you could visit me in the hospital?
                              FB Status 12:11 a.m. May 28, 2010.

I didn't want to be alone in the hospital. Again, as I look back, I was crying out for others to visit me while I was hospitalized. Why didn't I ask someone directly? With all the people and connections that I had, I didn't take the risk to say directly to anyone, "Please, come visit me in the hospital. I don't want to be alone." I also didn't want to be a burden to anyone. It can be so hard to take these sorts of risks in life. As I learned later on, taking risks was going to be something that I did very commonly. I would later learn to be a new person and that even through the fears, I would decide to speak my authentic voice. I would ask for what I needed, in spite of my fear of rejection. Eventually, a friend did offer to take my boys for a few days. I am forever grateful that she did. As it turned out, my recovery was tough and lasted much longer than I ever imagined. I didn't know it would be that way at the time. It's important that someone did help, because you never know how long a recovery will be. I was imagining that I would be one of the lucky ones that had a quick recovery. But, as it turned out, that had been a wrong estimation.

Six days until surgery. Went out with a few friends today and had a pedicure. I want the surgeon to look down at my feet and think how cute they look.
                              FB Status 3:18 p.m. May 29, 2010.

I know this may have sounded silly, but the truth is I had never had a pedicure until I was 40 years old. In fact, I think that's a reflection upon my own self-care. I didn't have the money to do these sorts of things, but even if I did, I still wouldn't have done it. In a way, I felt invisible throughout my life. Who needs to get a pedicure if you're invisible? I also didn't look down at my feet often, I am not sure I could have seen them. I imagined the surgeon performing the surgery and looking down at my pretty toes. As I think about it, there is no way he could have seen my toes because my feet were covered up during the surgery. Somehow it felt prettier to get a pedicure as I was spoiling myself before I went under the knife.

Amazing night skateboarding with dear friends. No I wasn't skateboarding, I know you weren't thinking that. My sons were. Five days until surgery. omg.

FB Status 11:54 p.m. May 29, 2010.

That night was a lot of fun. One of my sons loved skateboarding and going to the skate park was a regular night out for the family. One of my friends that I was with had the surgery herself. I felt comforted being with someone that knew what I would be experiencing in just five short days. We talked about the surgery and what to expect, and how everything would be changing real soon. I was grateful for someone who understood my concerns and fears.

Great day at church. God is good. Four more days until surgery. It's getting closer.

FB Status 10:45 p.m. May, 30 2010.

Countdown continues. At this point, there were only four more days to go. I didn't know how I could get through those next four days. In a way, it seemed like an eternity. In another way, it seemed to approaching much too fast. I was unprepared for that feeling. Today is the day that my doctor asked me to start a diet. The diet consisted of two protein drinks; one for breakfast and one for lunch. I was allowed one small dinner in the evening. This is when things really started to change for me. I am not sure if you are aware of it, but eating can keep feelings at bay. Once you stop eating excessively long enough, those feelings catch up to you. I knew that was going to happen. I began to get scared of emotions that I knew would show up.

We had an event planned with my church. It was a barbeque. On the drive to the barbeque, I became moody. I already was on the diet and my emotions were beginning to show themselves. In fact, I remember getting into an argument with the children.

I didn't feel like a very nice person. I know I was displacing my feelings, my fears and anxiety about the upcoming event, on my children. I felt like I stepped onto a rollercoaster. It was a new type of rollercoaster, an emotional one. Not to mention, I was attending a barbeque that evening, and I knew that I couldn't eat what they were eating. In fact, I didn't even want to go, but my children did, so I went.

I sat there awkwardly, not eating while everyone else consumed all around me. I was jealous and uncomfortable. Silently, I began to cry. No one knew that at the time. It was so loud and there was so much commotion going on at that time, that I was able to hide it from the people around me. I began to wonder how I would deal with these emotions as they became more prevalent, which was bound to happen after the surgery. That was an intense evening for me. I felt lonely and isolated and I wished in a way that others could see through my mask.

Emotions have begun to hit me. Would appreciate prayer for my emotions to stay balanced. Three more days until surgery.
FB Status 5:00 p.m. May 31, 2010.

How am I going to be able to handle the surgery and the emotions that come with that if I can't handle the emotions before the surgery? Frankly I can't even think straight, my head feels so cloudy.
FB Status 10:03 p.m. May 31, 2010.

So many people posted on this status about how proud they were of me, and that they were praying for me. I didn't feel as alone as I previously had felt. Maybe someone will visit me in the hospital is what I began to wonder. Maybe it's better to not create an expectation, as that can be a planned resentment. Either way, I knew people loved me and that was a good thing.

Great day today. Emotions back in check, someone must have been praying, thank you. Kids had a great time at the skate park, especially watching me figure out how to get the keys out of the trunk. Don't ask. Two more days until surgery.

FB Status June 1, 2010

Journal Entry #2:
Believe it or not I locked my keys in the trunk. Maybe I wasn't able to think as clearly as I thought I could. The Automobile Club came to my rescue that evening.

There is only one more day until my surgery. Well, to be more precise; one and a half days at this moment. I know you guys will miss me while I am gone. Or, it is entirely possible that you won't even notice I am gone. Either way, I appreciate the support.

FB Status June 2, 2010

Wow, I just read that statement I made publicly. Obviously, a part of me was wondering if anyone was really out there; if anyone really cared. I feel sad for the person that I was and the feelings she had at that time. She didn't know how to speak in a direct fashion about what she was feeling. I know that my emotions were definitely all over the place for me to be able to write that. I missed eating and stuffing my feelings, which is natural for an addict to miss their addiction. Yes, food can be an addiction much like drugs and alcohol. It's difficult to let go of a coping skill that you have been using for years. We all have to eat for sustenance. However, now I had to eat in balance. For me, that is not easy to do.

Many doctors require patients to diet for quite a while before their surgery date. This shows they are committed to the process of losing weight and also helps them to be as healthy as possible prior to the surgery. My doctor didn't require me to lose much weight. He recommended a small window of weight loss right before the surgery to kick-start my weight loss. My target weight loss was not as high as some of his other patients, so he made it simpler for me. Every doctor decides for their patients what their recommendations are. This is something you and the doctor decide together, so I can't speak to what your doctor will tell you.

> *Today is the surgery prep day, don't ask! Tomorrow I will be at the hospital. See you all soon.*
> FB Status June 3, 2010

"Don't ask," okay let me explain that one. The day before the surgery (at home) I drank some wonderful liquid, that tasted horrible, that prepared me for the surgery for the following day. Let's just say that I am pretty sure there was nothing left inside of me. I stayed close to the bathroom that entire day.

The next day was fairly planned out. A friend would be taking me to the hospital and keeping the children for a while. She and I had surgery exactly one year to the day apart from each other. She stayed by my side until they came to take me away for the surgery. After many years of struggling with my weight, many months of fighting to be approved for the surgery, and many days of pre-surgery preparation, I went to sleep knowing tomorrow everything would change.

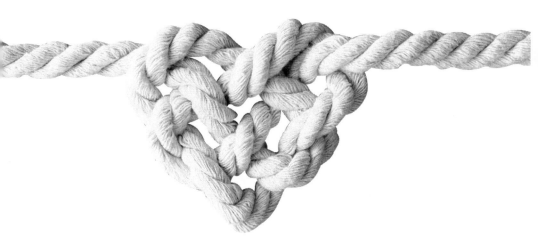

CHAPTER THREE

Surgery and the First Days of Recovery

Omg today is the day, I hope that I get into surgery fairly quick.
I have to be there at 1pm but I don't know when my surgery is.
FB Status - June 4, 2010

I am writing this a while after the surgery. I certainly wasn't up to documenting this at the time. I didn't go into surgery until late. The doctor was behind on his schedule. I am not sure why, but I believe another patient took longer in surgery than was expected. I waited for hours past the appointed time. As it turned out, I was the last patient of the day. Finally, I went in about 6:00 p.m. and came out of surgery around 8:30 p.m. The first thing I remember is being in a hospital room, with a nurse attending to my needs.

I felt horrible, which of course is understandable, I just had my insides re-plumbed. I was in a great deal of pain and in the beginning there seemed to be no relief in sight. I definitely don't do well with medications. I would take no medication, ever, if I could get away with it. I was offered pain medication, which made me sick and didn't help the pain. I was offered another pain medication, which also didn't help the pain and made me sick. After that, I refused those medications. I know lots of people would be thrilled with the opportunity to have medication at the press of a button. Not me, at least not those medications. I knew that there was another medication that usually helped me. I can't remember its name, but I believe it was a much milder drug. Anyway, they gave me the new medication. Instantly, I felt better. I remained on that medication while I was in the hospital. I did run into a little difficulty with getting my oxygen rate up. I have asthma, so I am not sure if that was the problem, but I couldn't seem to get enough air in my lungs. They told me if I couldn't get my oxygen rate up, I couldn't go home. I wanted to go home as quickly as possible. I started to write my FB statuses what was going on with my oxygen rate so that people would pray for me to feel better.

> *Second day in hospital. I need to get my breathing rate up or I can't go home tomorrow. Please pray.*
> FB Status June 5, 2010

> *I was able to more than double my oxygen rate in the last hour. Thank you for the prayer.*
> FB Status 9:32 p.m. June 5, 2010

During my hospital stay they were giving me a wonderful diet of tea, coffee, (I don't know why), and broth. I really wasn't hungry. Not a thing sounded good. I remember feeling some depression, some of which could have been partially due to the medication and because I was alone—except for the wonderful staff at the hospital. Apparently, I was good enough to be discharged so I called a friend to pick me up. My daughter remained behind to help with my recovery. I really can't thank her enough. I know I wasn't the easiest patient to deal with for the next week or so.

I am home. I made it out of there in a little more than 2½days. Clearly all the prayer has made a huge difference in my healing. Thank you so much. I am going to heal at home from here on.
FB Status 5:08 June 6, 2010

I was glad to be recovering at home. Hospitals are not a fun place to recover in. I know they are supposed to help us rest, which is difficult when the staff is coming in every few hours with a needle in their hand or to check on one thing or another. Just when I felt that I could fall asleep again, it seemed like they were coming back in my room, once again. Not only did they constantly check my blood pressure, they also continued to ask me to breathe into this strange device to prove that my lung capacity was up to par. I really didn't feel equipped, due to the asthma, to meet their medical standards quickly enough. There were a few other requests from the nurses, i.e. going to the bathroom before I was released. I guess I met their requirements because I made it home.

Hard night, last night. I need to get this drainage tube out, the weight of it is causing me soooooo much pain.
FB Status 7:41 a.m. June 7, 2010

Journal Entry #3:
This recovery is much harder than I imagined. Wait until you see my video during this period of time. I was trying to hold back from showing the pain that I felt, but honestly I didn't know how much more I could handle. I am taking the pain medication that they sent home with me, it's in a liquid form, which by the way tastes absolutely horrible. Then again, I am scared to take pills. I always kind of was, but now I am scared that something is going to get stuck in my pouch and that I will have even more pain. To get out of bed from a flat position is excruciating, it seems all I do is take a swig of the pain medication and try and sleep.

I need to go back to the doctor's office and get them to take out this tube. Every time I move, I can feel it moving in my organs. I don't remember anyone describing this kind of discomfort after their surgery. Why do I have to be the one the experiences pain so much worse? Not-to-mention the taste of the pain medicine is just awful.

To be fair, everyone has their own personal experience. I have since heard that many people describe that they transitioned easily from the hospital to home. I have heard other stories that had greater complications than what I experienced. There is no real way of knowing what your experience will be. It's a personal one and you will have your own story to tell. It's just like having a baby; we experience every birth in a different way.

Well I got someone to drive me to the doctor thank God and the drainage tube was taken out around 2 p.m., I feel like a new woman. I was scared it was going to hurt and it was completely painless and quite a relief. As soon as I came home, I passed out for hours. I woke up to my daughter being a little bored. I guess am not the best company for a 15 year old girl. I need to find a way for her to get out of the house. I can't drive her. Maybe a friend can get her out of the house for a while.
FB Status 8:56pm June 7, 2010

I had a hard time last night. Why does the pain hurt so much more at night?
I am not quite ready for my boys to come home, for some reason. Maybe their hyperactivity, they have a lot of energy. Thank you so much for all the support. It means so much to the kids and me. Love, Carol
FB Status 10:31 a.m. June 8, 2010

My friend brought me some more supplies, and gave my daughter a break for a few minutes. My friend tried to find me something that I could drink; a diet Snapple in a flavor that I could stand. She also took my daughter to get something to eat. Fast food. I am very grateful that my friend gave my daughter a break for a while. I felt a lot of guilt that I was putting her through so much because she was the one that was taking care of me.

I am much more mobile at this point and able to take care of some of my basic needs. Although I don't think I could have been alone for an extended period of time at this point, I could stand for a few minutes. I was also able to lie down in the bed easily. Sitting was not my favorite thing to do quite yet. I had no appetite at this point and no desire to eat or drink, which is not good. I needed to have nutrition and didn't know how to make myself have a desire to eat or drink. Water felt like a heavy weight when I drank it. I resorted to chewing on ice and eating popsicles for nutrition. I was dropping weight rapidly. It's hard to say how much weight I had lost, because my scale and the hospital scale were not in sync. It felt like I was dropping weight crazy fast. I know I had lost at least twenty pounds at this point. See Appendix B for weight loss statistics.

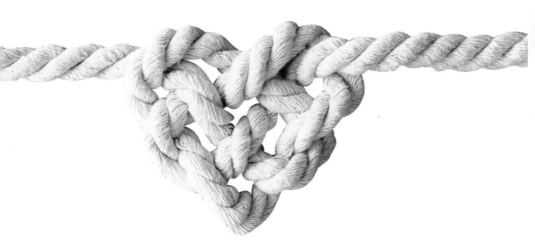

CHAPTER FOUR

Hanging in There

Hanging in there. Last three days have been rough. I think I am finely on the other side toward mending. My boys come back tomorrow. I guess it's time to get some meals in place for them.

FB Status, 12:28 a.m. June 11, 2010

Journal Entry #4:

I sure miss my sons, but am scared that I am in no position to take care of them. I do have more energy than before, which is weird. It's just that I don't have strength yet. I keep trying to drink water and it hurts so much whenever I take even a small sip. It feels like a bomb has gone off in my stomach when it goes down. Nobody has mentioned anything like that to me. Seriously am I the weirdest person on the planet? My reactions always appear to be so much more different than others' reactions.

My sons came home today, and it turned into a disaster. It was like PMS times ten. I totally lost it. I yelled at the kids. All I have been able to eat is popsicles and they ate them all. It's not like I can go to the store and replace them. I just lost it. I cried and cried and my friend came back and got the kids. I was not ready to deal with being a mommy yet.

FB Status 10:30 p.m. June 11, 2010

Of course as I read this now, I know that what was really happening was that I quit taking my medications without my doctor's approval and I sent myself into a tailspin of withdrawal. I should have gone off of my medications gradually, over a period of time, with a doctor's instructions. Instead, I decided in my stubborn way to just let go of all my medications from the moment that I got out of the hospital. This was a huge mistake and something I had to apologize to my children many times over for. Kids, again, I am still sorry for my behavior during that day. I was wrong and I than you that you were willing to accept my apology. I didn't mean to scare you guys.

What I didn't think about at this stage was that I had taken myself off all my prescribed medication. That was dangerous. Who am I to make a decision on what medication I should take? I just wanted off of them so bad, that I made the wrong decision and I was paying for it, or I should say my kids were. What I didn't think about was that when you are on medication you have to seek a doctor's advice on how to get off of them, i.e. step down the dosage until you can get completely off the medication. However, I am so stubborn. I have to do things my way and now I realize that. What I didn't realize at the time was that when you get off of medication improperly, it can take you on a wild ride of emotions.

I also think I was going through many other things at that time that were affecting my mood. Simply not eating can affect your moods. Ever seen someone grouchy that hasn't eaten? I'm just saying that many things were creating the perfect storm for me.

Journal Entry #5:

It's June 11th, it's been a week past my surgery date, exactly a week tonight, and last I checked I lost 24 pounds. This has been a hard recovery. I have never quite experienced anything like this. I still have a lot of pain. Thought I would go ahead and journal about my experiences and video blog each week as I am losing weight.

Week One: I can barely eat; I decided to stay on clear liquids this week. It works best for me. So I am mostly doing popsicles with a little broth. Many days the only thing I eat is 1-3 popsicles with a little broth and many days the only thing I eat is 1-3 popsicles. I know I am supposed to be doing protein, like in the protein pops, but omg those taste so bad I can't even say. I don't understand how anyone can drink those or lick those. I put mine in my freezer and after two licks and I couldn't do it.

Anyway, this pain is really getting to me. Why do I have to always feel more intense reactions than other people do? I have heard of people that didn't feel any pain after their surgery. I was in so much pain in the hospital that I was constantly trying to find relief. The hospital staff did offer me many different options. None of those worked for me, they just made me sick. They finally gave me something that was way less potent and it did the trick. However, since I came home, I was in so much pain that I could barely get up from bed. When I attempted, it pulled at the incision site and caused way too much pain. I just hope this stops soon. This can't go on for much longer, right?

Journal Entry #6:
My daughter is home alone taking care of me. I feel guilty that she is carrying so much of this burden at 15 years old, but what can I do? There is no one else to help. My boys are staying with a friend, thank God, as I don't feel capable of taking care of them. My sense of humor is completely gone. I started doing video blogs and I look so horrible on them. It doesn't help that I am sooo not comfortable in front of a camera, but you can also see how truly hard this is for me. I have seen other video blogs on YouTube. It seemed they looked great right away. I wonder if it's

my age or the fact that my body doesn't respond to things in the same way that the majority of the population does. When I had a surgery and the surgeon accidentally cut a main artery that is normally not placed there in most people and I decompensated (is this the right word???) quickly. Only if I was just like the average person, but to no avail, God has created me as I am, and I need to embrace the differences in me.

Omg, first relief from pain since my surgery.

FB Status 5:51 p.m. June 12, 2010

Journal Entry #7:

It's the eighth day past my surgery and the pain has been really bad. Finally, I was able to talk to the surgeon today and it turns out that the pain is not going away because the muscles in my stomach were being affected by the surgery. I just need to be patient and wait a little while and I will feel better. He instructed on what to take and how to take it and I am waiting to see if it finally gives me the relief that I need. I think it is, I don't know, I just took the medications few minutes ago and I am feeling a little better. I have lost 26 pounds already, I am 198, and so I am definitely on my way. I am feeling more awake, my sleep apnea is better, I don't know if it is completely gone but it's definitely close. I am actually awake in the daytime and not craving sleep. I am very emotional; I have had emotional ups and downs nonstop. I realized today that I don't even remember the last time I took my depression medication. I am going to get on that so I can get my hormones straightened out, because of course, I am dealing with my menstrual cycle as well. I have decided to keep doing these blogs because it is good for me, very cathartic and it helps me to be reflective in this process.

I am wondering if I am lactose intolerant now. I have never had any difficulty with dairy products, but I tried a little milk and I felt very strange. Like I felt my stomach gurgling and it just instantly felt odd. So I guess I won't be trying that for a while. However, I feel like I need to eat. My daughter made me a deviled egg, boy was that a huge mistake. What was I thinking? I think it was just way too rich and I felt like I was going to die for a few minutes. Okay I know I am being overly dramatic, but I certainly don't want to be doing that for a long time again. I know that I am really being a pain in the butt as a patient right now. I realize that I am expecting the world to revolve around me because I am not feeling well and I am being overly irritable. I know when someone is sick they can be this way, but I also know that this is wrong and I have to snap myself out of it, being irritable just isn't ok.

All I can say is please see your doctor, nurse or a nutritionist to help you with your diet during this stage, as each doctor suggests their own dietary plan.

It's June 13th, I feel a million times better. I was able to walk on my treadmill for five minutes today and go to the grocery store. I have one little problem, I am leaking at one of my suture sites and I just checked it, it looks horrible. Please pray that it heals up ASAP and doesn't get infected. I have been there before; don't ever want to go back.

FB Status 9:21 p.m. June 13, 2010

Journal Entry #8:
I am so glad that I am beginning to feel human. I am tired. Geez, I don't eat so that shouldn't be too surprising. However, I really did get on the treadmill for a few minutes today and I actually walked around the grocery store. I am so glad that I have really turned the corner; everything is going to get better every day from here. Yeah!!! The only thing is that yucky stuff is coming out of my suture sites. I have to keep cleaning up the

bandages. I am a little worried that this could mean something not good. I guess it is getting time to call the doctor and go see them.

I never talked to the doctor about stopping my medications. I was embarrassed to tell him. I tried to take one of the medications and didn't account for the fact that the dosage was now too high for me and I was horribly nauseous and dizzy for days. All the more reason to not tell anyone what I had chosen to do, it was completely embarrassing. Although it had taught me to never be my own doctor again.

Journal Entry #9:

My surgery was nine days ago. I am doing way better, even though I do have some seepage from one of my areas. I will have to call the doctor about that tomorrow. I have lost 28 pounds and I am 196. At this point, if I can lose 75 pounds more, that would be really great. So, I'm doing better and feeling better. I got on my jogger for the first time and walked for five minutes. I am going to try and to this throughout the day. Also, I will be putting away my own laundry and start to get my mail taken care of. My sons are coming back today. I wonder if I will be able to take care of the kids. I definitely feel better, but I am not myself by any means. I still feel irritable, hungry, and generally not me. I wonder what they will think about the changes in me.

Hi guys, doing great today. Still leaking, but as I found out, that is totally normal. Surgery was almost 10 days ago, today I'll try to drive. If you need to know where I am going so you can avoid me, just let me know!

FB Status 11:56 a.m. June 14, 2010

Journal Entry #10:

Today is ten days past my surgery date. I am becoming a Food Network addict. This new addiction cracks me up; now that I can't eat I am addicted to watching others cook! I am anxious to cook for my family even though I can't eat the food. I am a frustrated chef and I never realized how much. My clothes are already starting to hang on me. I already stopped wearing my first new set of underwear. Woo-hoo! So that is awesome and people are starting to come to see me. They really say my complexion looks different!

My boys came home yesterday and they were like "wow Mom you look so different already!" So I guess my goal at this point (I am just going to say 120 lbs. is my goal weight) would be 75 pounds away. It would be crazy if I could do that, I mean crazy! I am planning on doing a lot of getting up and around today. I am going to cook for my family today. Even though right now I am still really on a liquid diet; I haven't had the nerve to eat or drink anything else. Might try some scrambled eggs today, not sure. Or I might try some tilapia, something really soft. I also need to start cooking for myself. I know more of what I like and don't like. It doesn't matter to me right now, but what does matter is that I keep moving forward and keep healing.

My newfound joy in cooking is experimenting with what I can and can't eat. I'm sure this is something that you will be doing as well. Food preferences are subjective.

Journal Entry #11:

Well, I cooked a meal for the family. I was exhausted pretty quickly. What I didn't realize was that I can't even lick my fingers right now with the food that I am preparing for them. It is so second nature to lick as I go and taste test the food. I can't do that. So, I have to trust someone else's palette to taste the food and tell me what it needs. That is very frustrating. Plus nothing tastes the same anymore, so I don't think I can even judge what it tastes like for others. It's difficult to describe how food tastes different. Even many years later, food still tastes different than it did on the day of the surgery.[2] It did feel good to make the food and for my family to enjoy it. Could it be that I am closer to being myself again?

Went to a graduation ceremony today. Someone reminded me that I am not super woman yet. I kinda, well definitely over did it today. From now on, if I am gone from my house for a while I have to bring a cooler with cold water. I need to stay hydrated.

FB Status, 1:17 p.m. June 15, 2010

Journal Entry #12:

I don't know what I was thinking. I was not ready to be out in the hot sun quite yet. However, I really wanted to go support this graduate, and so I went. I did ok until right in the middle of the ceremony, I realized my menstrual cycle had started. I know no one really wants to know this, however it was my first since the surgery and it kicked my butt. Lots of pain, lots of other stuff and it began to make the day rather difficult. Then I realized that I felt dehydrated and I had nothing to drink. I really needed to prepare better. Not only that, but I was driving my three children home and I wasn't sure that I could do it. Thank God for my children, they kept urging me on during the whole trip telling me I could do it and before you know it, we were all home safe and sound. Next time I'll prepare better.

When I got home, I asked my daughter to make me some tomato soup. It sounded good and simple on my stomach. Not so much. Today was my first experience with "dumping", it happened within about 1-2 minutes of trying to drink a couple of sips. Boy, I don't want that to happen again. Maybe I shouldn't have had the tomato soup.

It just felt funny and I knew that if I didn't stop at that moment, I would throw up, dump or something. Either way, I knew it was my body's new way of saying to stop eating what you are eating. So I obeyed.

On top of that, I was having a real problem with my sutures. They were coming out of my body, like I needed to pull the strings as they are trying to get out on their own. This was weird, was this normal? I know I have always struggled with things staying in my body. When I broke my ankle, the pain from the metal that was left inside my body was so bad that I had to have another surgery to have it removed. What about my staples? Could they come out? Seriously, I have the weirdest body.

I did a mile on my treadmill today, it took two sessions and nearly 30 minutes, but I did it. Yeah for me.
FB Status 4:39 p.m. June 16, 2010

I already feel like I am beginning to have a new life. It's only been 12 days since my surgery, and yet in some ways I have more energy than I have had in many years. Of course, it helps to have lost some weight. But, this energy thing is something I was unprepared for. I used to sleep about sixteen hours a day; six of those in the daytime taking naps and waking up just as tired as when I went to sleep. Now I sleep six to eight hours and I wake up refreshed with energy. I feel so much better.

Journal Entry #13:
Ah June 16th, I have lost 31 pounds. It's a hard day in the sense that I am dealing with female issues. On the other hand, I was able to get on the treadmill today and I did a whole mile. I did it in two spurts. It took me almost 30 minutes to do it, but I did

it! I am going to shoot for 1 ¼ miles tomorrow. I don't care how many times it takes me to do it to get there.

On the other hand, when I go out, I get drained quickly and really don't feel like I should be driving yet, However, you've got to do what you've go to do. I needed to take the kids to church tonight. Tomorrow morning is my almost two week doctor's appointment. I am anxious to see what they say. I am still draining from surgical site and it's frustrating because it's not healing so I will see what they say when they check it out. My clothes are getting a little tiny bit loose after losing 31 pounds. However, I don't think it will affect my clothes much until I am probably at 50 pounds or so, but coming along, doing ok, and feeling better every day.

I am very grumpy, but I think a lot of that is my pain. Once the pain mellows out, it will help a lot. I don't know. I would love to see all this fat out of my face. I have been seeing the videos of people on YouTube; watching them lose their weight. When they lose the weight in their face, it is so amazing! I think I would look ok for an almost 50-year-old woman. I am really glad I did the surgery! I am just anxious for my body to adjust to the place where I could just get something down beyond popsicles! That is still pretty much all I am taking in right now.

It's important to understand that moodiness may ensue as your body's fat cells dump your hormones into your blood stream causing a hormonal imbalance. There are many studies that have been done on this phenomenon. I know for myself, I had about six weeks of extreme moodiness as the hormones were released into my body. That is not something I would ever like to experience again. The good news is that once I lost a lot of weight in the beginning of the process, I didn't experience that again.[3]

Journal Entry #14:

It is June 17th. Today is 13 days past my surgery. I have lost 32 pounds so far. I went to the doctor today. They say I may have a pre-infection, but they aren't sure. They put me on antibiotics, but I haven't been able to take them yet because my stomach is still such a mess. What else? I'm doing pretty good with my kids and I did 1.2 miles today on the jogger. I did it just a little bit past 30 minutes so I am going to try and stick to that 30 minute time frame for now, and do it daily. I can't wait to do this thing when I am not lying down with pain in my belly still, but I got myself to the doctor and back, and then to the store with Dylan and got everything I needed. Picked up my prescription, and then passed out from sheer exhaustion. So I am 192 pounds now and I have lost 32 pounds.

So back to this pre-infection. My doctor made a big deal about the leaking. He shoved his fingers all around the suture sites! By the way, it hurt like heck! Felt like he was shoving his fingers throughout my organs. I guess what he was doing was trying to seep as much liquid out of me as possible. Boy I don't want to do that all over again. Although I am glad because at least most of the liquid is out of me and there is less chance of an infection. I wonder if I will stop leaking now. Did he do something magically that will stop that? Seriously, I have heard of no one having this problem, except for me.

I know as I am saying this, someone is reading this and saying, "Hey! Wait, that happened to me, too." I'm sorry that it happened to you, too. However, I am glad I'm not completely alone in the weird body category, if you know what I mean.

I'm still leaking from one of my sutures. If you think of it I could use your prayer, this is really getting annoying, it hasn't healed for two weeks plus it hurts.

FB Status 11:25 p.m. June 18, 2010

Journal Entry #15:

It's exactly two weeks since my surgery now, two weeks tonight and I have lost, hold on, 34 pounds. My goal is getting closer. I haven't been lower than 160 in years and years and years, and I can see that possibility in sight. I can't remember being that size as an adult. If I think about it, maybe I was that weight as a child. I'm still not eating enough. I had two popsicles today, some water, and nothing else. Didn't exercise and was able to sleep a lot during the day. Still leaking from my site, getting tired of this, having to change this gauze twice a day and it is pretty saturated. This has been going on for over a week.

I am so glad that I have been keeping up with this journey electronically, i.e. Facebook and video blogging. It definitely helps me to keep clear in my head how this journey has gone for me. I have to say that I have been having a lot of fears lately. One of my fears is dumping. I have only dumped one time, I think right after I had that tomato soup. I had tomato soup again a few days later but it wasn't a problem the second time. It is so not fun having to be very careful about what, when and how I eat. Another fear I have is that I would stretch my pouch and gain the weight back again. I know that if I was to start drinking carbonated beverages, this could acerbate this stretching and my weight loss could stall. I don't intend on drinking soda ever.[4]

After all I have been through since this surgery, I certainly don't want that to ever happen. Although at this stage it is really hard to imagine. My other fear is that something would get stuck in my pouch. I have heard horror stories about people that ate something and it got stuck and they had to go to the emergency room to get help. Geez, I pray that won't happen to me ever. I know that there are definitely no guarantees in that.[5]

Leaking has diminished for the first time, yeah. I am praying
that it will stop completely. Thanks for your prayers.

FB Status 10:56 p.m. June 20, 2010

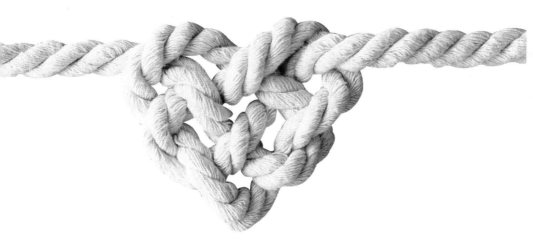

CHAPTER FIVE

Healing Continues at a Faster Rate

Journal Entry #16:

It's two weeks and two days past my surgery date. I have lost 34 pounds, nothing in the last couple of days. I exercised 1.32 miles yesterday. It took three times in 10 minute intervals to get it done. I feel weaker. I now that I am not eating enough protein. Protein is so important to anyone that has been through a surgery and I am failing in this area.[6]

Journal Entry #17:

It is 18 days past my surgery date. I am eating better; I have been able to eat soups every day. I have been completing many errands everyday and that's good! It shows that my energy is remaining at a good place. I am still not as responsible with my protein as I should be. My incision is still leaking. Yesterday it leaked everywhere and I almost threw up! I'm frustrated with that. Here it is 2 ½ weeks post-surgery. This has been going on for a week and a half. I'm beginning to wonder if it is every going to stop. I am going to try to go to San Diego with some friends because someone else is getting ready for her gastric bypass and I thought it would be nice to support her. I think I might be losing inches and haven't really realized it because this last week has been a little hard. I still have this huge chin.

L et's talk about this for a minute. I think that we all get fixated on different body parts when we are going through this process. You may want your stomach to get smaller. Someone else wants their double chin to go away. I have seen others that super focus on their legs. Everyone has their different areas that they would like to see tightened up on their body when they are losing weight. For me that is my chin.

Journal Entry #17 (continued)
I am so obsessed with my double or triple chin. I look at it every day. Especially when I am videotaping, there is no way to get away from that. I can't wait for that to disappear.

There is a mental condition that is called Body Dysmorphic Disorder that we as therapists see from time to time. This condition is where the individual may be preoccupied with nonexistent or slight defects or flaws in their physical appearance.[7] I can't wait until I work through my disconnection between my body image as it changes and I become a new me. I know that this takes time to line up both physically and emotionally.

Journal Entry #18:
It's June 26th, about three weeks since my surgery. I have been struggling with a plateau for the last five days because I haven't lost a pound. That is very frustrating and it's very easy to begin to think this magic pill is no longer working when you don't lose weight for that long. However, you have to realize that at times your body is not ready to let go of more weight and it's helpful to look at your pattern thus far to see that you will soon reach your next goal. Don't lose hope at this point. I know for me I disconnected somewhat from this blogging process for those days when I didn't feel I had successes to share. The good news is that I lost two more pounds as of this morning. So, that makes me 38 pounds down. I am still leaking, but it seems to be slowing

down. I am really hoping that it is starting to heal, but I am not really sure. I am noticing my chin is getting a little better, I mean my chins, my many, many chins.

I drove to San Diego yesterday to help my friend who was completing some of her pre-surgical process. The important part of that statement was that I drove. It's approximately two hours away from my house, and I couldn't tell you the last time I drove that far. I would never have attempted driving this far in the past. I would have been afraid that I would have fallen asleep or needed to take a break along the way, it wouldn't have been possible. Instead this was a fun trip, taken with two friends, all of which have either had the surgery or were going to have the surgery. This has become a new circle of friends for me, those of us that support each other through our recovery. I never imagined that I would already be helping others, giving them hope and helping them understand the trials and tribulations that they will experience before, during and after their surgical procedure.

I will discuss this further, when I share about the support groups later in the book.

I have been eating protein for the last 3 days. I have been eating salmon cooked in olive oil with some dill. I ate a Baby Bell and then I had some smoked salmon. I am eating natural protein. What are you eating at this stage? Whatever you are eating, remember every one of us is directed according to our doctor's Dietary Plan. You don't need to be eating what I am eating. You need to eat what is best for your body. You will figure this out in time. Be kind with yourself and know that which foods work for you will make sense over time.

Journal Entry #19:

Tomorrow will be one month since my surgery. I have lost 42 pounds so far. Wow! I have lost 42 pounds so far! Let me sit in this and revel before moving on.

I think that it is important for us to take those moments to honor what we have accomplished. It is so easy for us to get caught up in the numbers. The numbers we usually are caught up in, is our goal, not how far we have come. Remember, this whole process is just that. It is a journey and I can't begin to tell you how that journey morphed from the physical to the emotional back and forth for some time to come. Keep honoring those precious moments that happen along the way. Recognize that your process is in exactly the place that it is supposed to be. I am beginning to let go of a lot of clothing. You may find yourself struggling in this area. I have seen so many others struggle in letting go of baggy clothing. It's difficult to recognize that it's time to let go of big sizes. There is a mental adjustment to the clothes being too big. There may also be an adjustment to the fact that your pocketbook needs to keep buying clothes to keep up with your weight loss. I often recommend to others to use both "hand-me-downs" and thrift stores as options during the time that you are quickly losing weight. There were times I was changing sizes almost every two weeks. I confess there were times I bought things and returned them before I ever had the chance to wear them because I lost sizes so fast. It is ok. When the time comes to let go of your bigger clothing, they can be of use to other friends going through the surgery or by donating to your local community.

You know I haven't felt that I could work for years now. It used to be that I had some energy. The sleep apnea killed that. I was tired 24/7. Not the normal tired you get to throughout the day. The closest thing that I could equate it to was pregnancy tired. Sorry men, if you are reading this part as you probably don't understand. When you are pregnant, there is a kind of tiredness that hits your body that is like nothing else. With my sleep apnea, I was tired 24/7. I guess I was not getting any restorative sleep. I was probably waking up throughout the night from snoring and not realizing it. So to me, I never really felt like I was awake for years. I don't know how I functioned. In fact, the kids and I went on a trip to Los Angeles during Easter Vacation this year. I was determined to find a way to have a good spring vacation for the kids even though I couldn't afford much. The story is that we were on a list for tickets to see the shows in Hollywood. We were sent tickets to see a pre-show event for the Kid's Choice Awards. I was planning on spending the night at the venue and hoping somehow there would be a miracle and we could get tickets for the big show as long as we got there early enough for the pre-show event. My children and I went out late at night, at 10 pm to the UCLA campus to spot out a place we could sleep. As the kids and I were trying to figure out what to do, a man came out of the main venue and asked how many tickets we needed, I said for me and the kids it was four tickets. He said do you have friends coming, I said yes; I have a friend and her family that is coming and my sister and her daughter and friend are coming as well. So this man handed me 18 free tickets for the Kid's Choice Awards! All he asked was that I didn't sell them on EBay. You can look up the worth of those tickets. What he gave us was a phenomenal gift. I, of course, agreed and took the tickets.

The next day, my friend came down with her family and my sister came with hers. We ended up with one ticket leftover that we eventually gave to someone at the event that was desperate to get a seat. In the meantime, we had all day to explore the city until the event that evening. We went to a few places including La Brea Tar Pits. While we were out, I fell asleep while the kids were in the museum of the Tar Pits. I always fell asleep wherever I went or I basically didn't even try to go anywhere. One of the kids snapped my picture while I was asleep. Here I thought I looked pretty in my purple shirt. What I really looked like was a beached whale. At least that's how I felt. How did I hide from the truth about how I looked? I was mad at the kids for snapping my picture because I was so embarrassed about how I looked on film. The truth was that it was a huge thing for me to be able to stay awake as long as I did for that full day. Driving through Los Angeles and trusting I could stay awake was a real faith thing for me. My days were like that every day. Now I can do so many things. I do nap occasionally, but before the surgery I woke up late; then took a nap around 1:00 or 2:00 p.m. That nap had to last three hours. Even then when I woke up, I was still sleepy. I remember I would do everything to not have to drop off and pick up the kids as I just didn't have the energy. I knew that was no way to live my life. I needed to be there for my children and I couldn't do it that way.

Anyway, I was talking about being unable to work. I was sleeping so many hours in a day that I couldn't stay awake long enough to work. I had to be able to support my children. I had to get a job. I just didn't know how to do that. I had become such a flake during this time because I couldn't function the way other people could. Back in the day, I was so responsible and always followed through. I can't wait until my life turns around and I am able to be the person that I know I can be; someone who is responsible and able to work.

Journal Entry #20:

It is July 8th. I have lost 46 pounds now. My weight is 178 and tomorrow will be five weeks since the surgery. The good news today is that I went to see my pain management specialist and he said that my Body Mass Index (BMI) has gone down from 43.4 to 33.2 in almost 5½ weeks which is awesome, totally, totally, totally, totally awesome! I can see some weight loss in my face but still have a double chin and to me my body looks pretty gross. Although I am wearing a lot smaller sizes, it's still not good enough. I am certainly not ready to meet any men. I have a long way to go through this. Not even sure if I want to date, I'm scared. Especially, think about the fact that I'm used to being invisible. You can't remain invisible and date. Those are mutually exclusive events. I'm still frustrated that I can't drink water. Ice chips are still my go to. I guess this process continues to be one day at a time, and I need to remain in the present for every day.

I have achieved 50% of my weight loss goal. Although I am beginning to notice that my energy is not as high as it was. I'm wondering if that's because I am losing weight so fast.

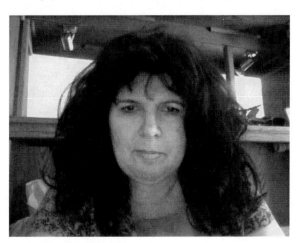

So the doctor tells me to drink 64 oz. of water a day. Why do I feel so dehydrated? I was ready to drive myself to the hospital to get fluids in me. Then I looked at the bottles I have been drinking, they are 9 fl oz. I was thinking I could drink 4 bottles and be fine, and yet I never even drank that much. Anyway I should have been drinking at least six. No wonder I was always nauseous—duh.

FB Status 3:12 p.m. July 18, 2010

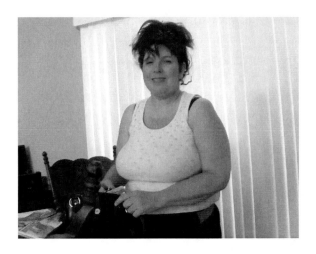

Journal Entry #21:

It is July 18th. I realized that I haven't videotaped myself in quite some time. Every time that I hit a plateau, it is hard for me to get in front of the camera or a piece of paper to write about my lack of success. I haven't lost weight in six days. However, I haven't gained weight in six days either. So why am I so hard on myself to think that I am now the very definition of a failure when my weight loss stalls? I know that our bodies let go of weight when they are ready to. It's so easy for me to define myself based on my weight.

This reminds me of my relationship with my mother. She was 80-90 pounds her entire life, until she was dying from cancer. During that phase of her life, she actually ballooned up to 126 pounds. I remember the horror she showed on her face when we weighed her and she saw that number. In fact, I can't remember a time when I visited my mother that she didn't say, hey you have gained weight, or hey you have lost weight. No wonder I was and still am so defined by what I weigh. My mom eventually weighed so little and was so frail that I estimated she had to be somewhere around 60-70 pounds. Thanks to cancer, she wasted away. She was a very tiny woman, only 5' tall. Her mother and my father's mother were even smaller than that. However, I digress.

As I am going through this process, my understanding of where my distorted body image came from, whether it was from media, my friends and or my upbringing, I seemed to define my worth by what the scale said. If the number was down, I felt valuable. If the number was up, I felt like a failure. The truth is that I was neither. That was just a number on a scale. A number doesn't convey who I am, what I have accomplished in my life, or what I will accomplish in the future. It doesn't declare that I am less than. It doesn't state that I am a kind and considerate person. It only conveys my weight. There are, of course, factors that come into play with my weight at this time. Ladies, you know if you are expecting your cycle you tend to gain a little weight, plus we fluctuate at any given moment throughout the day in our weight. All this to say, who cares that I haven't lost any weight in the last six days. All that means when I am plateauing, is that my body is getting ready to shed weight and take me down to a new normal.

One thing that I like to do is keep track of inches and not weight. I have lost weight so many times in the past and the number on the scale didn't move, but my body proportions changed throughout that time. It's like your body is being sculpted at a cellular level. If you are keeping track of your inches and sizing of clothes, that may help you to feel more of a success. Through this process I have noticed that one day my stomach seems smaller, or my hips are changing, or I am losing weight in my breasts. The weight doesn't come off in a consistent manner.

One other thing I am noticing is that as I continue to be dehydrated, I don't lose weight. I believe my body is fighting to keep as much of weight on as possible, as it may think I am in starvation mode. That is nature's way of protecting your body.[8]

Journal Entry #22:

I know that I need to be drinking so much more water than I am drinking. It is so frustrating to me, before my surgery my favorite drink was water, and now it is my least favorite drink. I have probably been drinking one fourth or less of the water I need to be drinking thus I have been very nauseated and not wanting to eat. I realized that I need to be very meticulous in counting how much I am drinking. My ability to focus is minimized currently and that is in direct correlation to my dehydration.[9]

Feeling way better today. My primary job right now, drink, drink, and drink water.

FB Status 9:12 a.m. July 19th, 2010

Journal Entry #23:

It is July 21st. It's been six weeks and five days since my surgery and I finally lost a pound. I hadn't lost anything in eight days. It's funny how we reach these weight loss plateaus where our body is simply unwilling to let us move on to the next stage. I was taught in a support group that increasing our water intake, increasing our protein intake and increasing our exercise intensity, are all ways in which to move past the plateau that we are stuck on.[10]

I am having some friends come to visit my family this week. They will be staying with us. They are from another country. I have always been a very spontaneous person; making friends around the world and inviting them to stay with us as an interesting experience. I met this friend when I was pregnant with my now eleven year old. We were on a list together of women pregnant with children in the same month. I have a fear about this visit. When we made our plans to visit each other I just assumed that I would be mostly healed from my surgery. As I am struggling with the dehydration, and no taste for eating, I am concerned that I won't be able to keep up with my friends while they are visiting. I guess I will find out soon enough if I miscalculated how ready I am to have company.

Journal Entry #24:
I am beginning to eat fish now. I know that I need to eat protein, and most protein is difficult for me to digest. I am experimenting with mild fish. I am trying everything to eat from tilapia, fresh tuna and sashimi --- you know, raw fish. For some reason raw fish is something that I crave now. I have lost 55 pounds, which is equal to about 56% of my weight loss. I am spending a lot of my time chastising myself. It honestly feels at times that I have a hammer and I am beating myself with it. I struggle with being kind to myself. It's time to learn to praise myself and to be proud of my accomplishments.

Have you ever heard of a critical parent?[11] It is that voice in your head that is telling you you are not good enough, who do you think you are, etc. those kinds of comments. That inner voice in my head keeps telling me I need to exercise more, do more, and do it better, or I will be a failure. I have spoken with countless people that have gone through this process that also have been their own worst critic. I am not saying that there can't be an exception, because there can be. However, if you are hearing that still, small voice in your head telling you to do better, try and remember that this is not unusual. Tell that voice to quiet down, that you are just where you need to be in this very moment.

So, the thoughts that cross my mind are: "When will I reach my goal?" "I should be losing more weight and much faster." "I should.......(fill in the dots)."

Try to remember, *shoulds* and *musts* are those negative thoughts that may cause us to feel less than. Then ask yourself when has a *should* and a *must* ever been beneficial to you? I dare you to think of a time that that has generally helped you to feel positive about a situation.

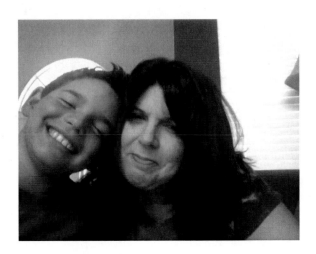

Journal Entry #25:

Alright, don't tease me. I signed up for eHarmony for one month just before my surgery date. This guy started writing me and telling me how we were meant to be together, he just felt it was from God. I told him, "If you feel that way, why don't I feel that way?" He seemed a bit desperate. Nevertheless, we have written each other for about three months now. He didn't know my weight, who brings that up? When we first started talking, I didn't tell him I was going into the hospital to have surgery. I finally told him that I had the surgery. I really didn't want him to know. Maybe it was a test to see if he would leave me alone after that. But to no avail, he continued communication with me. Anyway, we haven't talked on the phone, just written emails. So, at this point, I feel safe.

One day I started hearing this noise that sounded like water running in the house, and I realized that the downstairs bathroom floor was hot all the time. I really had no idea what that meant. Then, the gas company showed up and said that my gas usage was through the roof. I didn't understand. I rarely ever use gas unless I cook or do laundry. Anyway, it turned out that

I had a water leak. It was the hot water which was causing the gas and water bills to go up. So I called the eHarmony guy I had been writing to. I actually had never heard his voice until that moment. I was scared about the water leak and didn't want to be alone when the plumber came to give me his estimate. I doubt if this makes sense, I invite in a plumber that I don't know, and a man that I never met to be "the man" on the scene. I figured if he was a man he could tell me if the estimate sounds like an appropriate amount. I was so scared what the plumber was going to say it was going to cost to fix. However, I have a lot of weight to lose and didn't want him to see me yet. This guy (he shall remain unnamed, mostly because I forgot his name) came over and so did the plumber. It turned out it wasn't nearly as bad as I thought it was. Once I heard the good news, this guy took me out to eat. Geeze, I don't eat --- perfect first date. Well, I got some fresh tuna sashimi and ate a few bites. It was so good. A week later, I never saw that guy again. It didn't really matter, but I had to wonder what happened? Did he leave because I was still overweight and he assumed things would stay that way? Or maybe he left because at that point I smelled funny, almost like maple syrup because my body was in ketosis?

My doctor suggested remaining in ketosis the first 75% of my weight loss, which means eating protein primarily. When you primarily eat protein, this causes your pores to sweat out the toxins in your body. You, honest to God, smell like maple syrup. While he was at my house, the thought kept coming to mind to tell him what was really going on. I felt that nervous tension, like you and the person know that one of you has something to say, and it remains unsaid. I think of it as "cordial hypocrisy" or the "pink elephant in the room" that isn't being addressed. As I didn't have a clear authentic voice at that juncture, I chose to stay silent, and I never saw or heard from him again.[12]

I guess I will never know what happened with that one. I don't think that it is very important to know that answer anymore. I chalk that up to a funny story.

Journal Entry #26:

It is August 5th, which would make it two months and one day past my surgery date. I have lost 57 pounds. I have felt strange lately. For the last week or two, I have felt bigger than ever, of course, due to my menstrual cycle. My hormones are somewhat out of whack. In other words, my periods have been inconsistent.[13]

I think the real issue that I am experiencing, is that I am really coming out of denial about how big I really was. Like in my mind, I always looked like I look now. But the reality is, is that it took almost sixty pounds of weight loss to get where the vision I had of myself in my head was.

So clearly, I didn't look that way before and that's hard to realize that I was walking around at that higher weight and didn't even know it. Denial is a defense mechanism. It's a way of not believing something is true when it is. For now, I imagined myself thinner. Thus, in my mind, I was --- however, I wasn't. I look back and I feel arrogant that I was so out of touch with how I looked to others. At least that was the way I processed through those feelings; thinking who was I to think that I looked better than I did? That is why I still carry around with me, to this day, that last picture that was taken of me before the surgery. I felt super cute that day, and as I look at myself in that picture, that is not what I see.

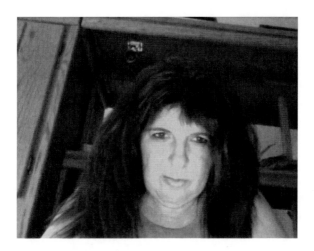

I believe this is the first glimpse of acceptance that I was experiencing. Through that process of acceptance, I began to grieve. I grieved for the woman that I am today and how her dreams have remained stagnant due to her weight. I grieved for so many things during that time. I cried. I spent a good deal of time in reflection. I wrote in my journal and began to come to terms with it all. Or, at least I had a glimpse of the beginning of all the steps of grieving that I would experience. It's not the weight that this is really about. It's the recognition of who I was and who I was becoming now. The weight is just a number that helps to quantify what I am feeling. I hope that makes sense to you, because this is the important stuff. It's all about grief. As a therapist, I learned an acronym D.A.B.D.A, which stands for Denial, Anger, Bargaining, Depression, and Acceptance. This is how grief works. It is not a linear process. You may start with denial, or any one of the other abbreviations, and you may ping pong back and forth experiencing each emotion, until eventually you end up with acceptance, or at least that is the end goal. There will be various stages of grief that you experience. Honor each step and allow yourself to be immersed in every feeling. Don't skip any one of them, as they are a specific formula that eventually leads to healing and an understanding of the new person that you are becoming.

During this time, I have been looking back at pictures of various memories and reminiscing about the past. I even have been looking at more current pictures, and thinking, I still have a billion pounds to lose. I know I am being harsh on myself; it's just sometimes I don't ever think I will get to my goal.

Journal Entry #27:

I am eating a little more now. My stomach can handle more than a few bites at a time. However, my hormones that have been stored in my fat cells keep coming out. This makes me experience a lot of depression --- well, definitely some depression. I am irritable, so that is some part of depression. Remember this is still a process and this will continue in the way that your body functions.

Just recently my church took some pictures of a group of people and as I looked at the group of people, I realized it still feels like I am the biggest person in the room. Not just my body stature, but also my face is also really big. Maybe that's one of those body image issues that I will struggle with for a while to come. I would just like to see myself smaller than at least one person in the room. Who am I kidding? I don't want to not notice my size at all. In a way I want to be invisible still.

The interesting thing is that as I lose weight, I am beginning to wear smaller sizes, but petite smaller sizes. That really messes with my head. How can I be in a petite, when I am still so overweight? I know, petite is about proportion and I could be very high weight and small at the same time. In fact, I was petite when I had a 50% BMI, and over one hundred pounds overweight. Although I tried on and bought a size 14 dress recently, it has been a long time since I could wear that size.

Journal Entry #28:

It's been more than two months since my surgery date and I am beginning to feel the weight of the world on my shoulders. As a single Mom, I am dealing with many different issues. Remember that leak in my house? Now it needs to be fixed. Shockingly enough, that requires money which I don't really have. I know that I need to get a job. Yet, I feel that I am still too tired to work. Being alone and problem solving isn't easy as a woman. Yet, I am not ready to date and wouldn't even consider that at the moment, if there was someone even interested in dating me. Also, I heard that soon enough my hair will start falling out due to the trauma from my surgery. It's not that I worry about hair loss. I have been told that I have enough hair for three people on my head. It's just one more change to process through. Maybe I will be one of those fortunate ones and my hair will remain intact.

Journal Entry #29:

Well it's two months and one week since the surgery. I have completed 62% of my weight loss goal. I am beginning to dream about eating all those carbohydrates that I haven't eaten in so long. And when I say dream, I mean it. There are times when I dream at night of eating cakes, donuts, burritos, pizza, and bread. Yes, I said bread. I am too scared to even think of trying bread. The funny thing is that I never really cared much about bread, but other people tell me that it is the one thing they miss the most. When I wake up from those dreams, I am in shock in a way, I feel like I cheated on my diet. Then I realize that I didn't cheat on my diet and I am still eating protein only. Bummer.

I have now accepted that guy I had been emailing with for three months is officially gone. I tried to text him a few times, maybe twice and then I let it go. In a way, I was sorry that I ever took the risk to call him in the first place to ask for his help. I was only looking for a friend. But that risk came with a great price. The pain I exposed myself to be the very emotions that had caused me to gain the weight in the first place. The weight was a protection. I wanted to be invisible. I wanted to not put myself out there and take a risk, because I didn't think I could manage the emotional aftermath. It worked, because I was morbidly obese. No one approached me, no one asked me out and thus I remained safe behind a wall of my own imprisonment.

Journal Entry #30:

I recently overcommitted to help a friend with her daughter's wedding. When I say that I overcommitted, I mean I really overcommitted. I was working long hours, and I was unequipped to do so. There were times that I felt ready to drop and I kept on helping. That was a mistake for me. This was the beginning of a deeper understanding of my codependent behaviors and my inability to say no when I was asked for help. I started to feel sick, not quite my self as well as more and more tired. I felt like my physical health was declining. Something was going wrong and I didn't know it yet. All I knew was that I should have said no and I didn't know how to do that, at least not yet.[16]

Journal Entry #31:

Guess what? I just found out that I have another water leak in the house. What the heck? I am beginning to wonder if I am the unluckiest person in the world. Ok, maybe a bit dramatic. Houses do require upkeep and I wasn't keeping up my house. So that's what happens.

I am continuing to lose weight. However, my double chin seems to have a life of its own. I don't think it is going anywhere. I am still fixated on that. Why can't I fixate on the positives? Is it due to the fact that no one taught me that skill? I have been trying to teach my children to notice those positives in their life; however it's difficult to teach what you don't have. People pay attention to your actions and not your words. I hope through this process that I become a much more positive person.

Journal Entry #32:

It's been 2 months and 2 weeks since my surgery and I have 30 pounds to go which is weird. It's really the lowest weight I have ever been. This makes me realize that I haven't been at a low enough weight all of my life, and I have been kidding myself that I was. While I was losing weight, my wardrobe has been disappearing piece by piece. I had a range of sizes in my closet from one size 4 to size 16 or 18. At least my collecting, let's not call that hoarding, of clothing, was beneficial in this process. I began to weed out the bigger sizes and when I filled a bag I donated it to whoever needed it, while I began to fit in some of the smaller sizes. I would say that I also shopped at thrift stores and occasionally at Kohl's. You know the place where you can put a sale with a coupon, a rewards card and get back credit to use the following week which starts the process all over again. I think my body is losing weight disproportionately. In other words, the top part of my body is losing weight quicker that the bottom.

My skin is still holding up fine, I want to get my teeth done. I am embarrassed by my teeth, that's why I don't smile in my videos.

That is one of my dreams, to have bright white teeth. My mother always said that she never drank milk during her pregnancy with me and my teeth came in yellow from day one. I also had a bit of a mishap when I was around age 8. Believe it or not, I was skating on wet cement and tripped and fell. My teeth hit the concrete. One of my front teeth died that day, although

I didn't realize it until many years later. A dentist finally told me that I would need to cap my front teeth, as they can't recover from an accident like that.

I want to take a moment and talk about this surgery. People say it's the easy way out. Nothing could be further from the truth.

This is probably the hardest thing that I have done in my life. I have given birth to three children, one without anesthesia taking effect. This process is painful, tiring, and exhilarating. I could use a million different descriptive words here. Many of us that go through this process all have a different story of the side effects that we have experienced. The effects will last, as far as I know, for the rest of my life.

I wouldn't say that was taking the easy way out. I would say that was making a hard choice that was difficult to make.

Because I have never been this weight before, I am really on new ground. I don't have a reference point in which to gauge what will happen from here. It really is a new season for me, a season that I can't envision, or see what it will look like.

Journal Entry #33:
I have lost 71% of my weight and I am beginning to experiment with adding in carbohydrates. I have already been eating everything. I have been doing that on and off for awhile. It's just that I barely eat anything, so I give myself permission to eat in order to meet my nutritional needs. Almost three months out, I expected. I know expectations are planned resentments, but I did expect to feel better. What is going on? I am moody and I am feeling alone. I have decided to call the doctor next week and see if I need to treat my depression medically. I wonder if losing weight this fast is affecting my mood.[17] I don't know if it's just the rapid weight loss that is causing some of this, the estrogen coming out of my fat cells, or what. I've lost seven pounds this week. That hasn't happened in a long time and still this double chin remains. My closet is getting more and more barren, approximately half the size it was before.

I made a protein shake, it wasn't too bad. I am going to get more protein in me.

FB Status 8:34 p.m. August 23, 2010

Journal Entry #34:
I am beginning to get closer to that all-important three month weight loss anniversary. I had a terrible experience yesterday. I took a trip to Oak Glen, a local area known for its apple picking, fresh pies, wonderful barbeques, hayrides etc. My children even learned to make a candle many years ago when we visited there. It's not too far away, about thirty minutes, although that can seem like a long time when you aren't feeling tip top. Anyway, we went into one of those lovely little stores that sell barbeque, coleslaw, corn, and nice little jars with quaint packaging. I ordered some coleslaw, but there must have been some sugar in it. I literally took a few bites and nearly went down for the count. My memory is foggy of that event. I laid down on the grass outside the shop and began to recover from, I don't know what.

The next problem was that I needed to drive my family back home and I didn't feel good. Thankfully, we were with friends and my dear friend took charge and drove my car home. I lost about 2½ pounds over night from that experience. I began to realize that I was also having other physical affects to my body. Next thing I knew was that my feet kept falling asleep and my hands were contorting in strange ways. You know when there is something wrong and you try and dismiss it and hope it will go away on its own. That thing called denial was working overtime in me at that time. I didn't want to believe that I was sick and needed help. It was time to go to the hospital.

"If you trade your authenticity for safety, you may experience the following: anxiety, depression, eating disorders, addiction, rage, blame, resentment, and inexplicable grief."

— Brené Brown

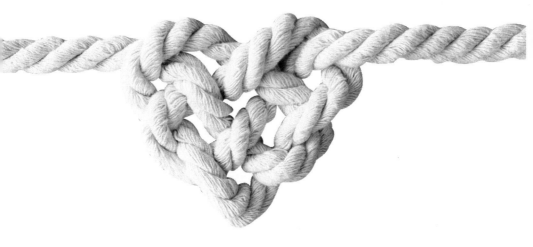

CHAPTER SIX
Back to the Hospital

Please keep the kids and me in your prayers. I am taking myself to the hospital in the morning. I know I am majorly dehydrated. I have tried everything to get myself back on track. I give up. I need help from a doctor. Hopefully they will just hydrate me and send me home, that is my prayer.

FB Status 12:34 a.m. August 28, 2010

Been in hospital all night. Problem is low potassium. Hope to be home by noon.

FB Status 8:49 a.m. August 28, 2010

(4 comments, 1 like)

Well I got home around 11:30am. I'm not going to pretend this was a fun hospital visit, although I am happy to know what has been wrong with me. My potassium level was 2.17, it's supposed to be 3.50 to 5.0. I thought I was dehydrated; instead I had an electrolyte imbalance. Anyway thanks for the support, my hands and feet are getting better already.

FB Status 4:24 p.m. August 28, 2010

I am sitting up and my head is clear, what a trip man, better than the best of drugs.
>FB Status 5:03 p.m. August 28, 2010

Today is a hard day. Getting enough potassium is proving to be difficult. I am sleeping most of the time. I get up, eat something with potassium in it, don't say bananas, apparently they don't have enough. Then I wait an hour, take a potassium supplement then fall back to sleep. I am processing feelings right now about how serious this really was. Thank you for all your support. Please keep me in prayer.
>FB Status 2:56 p.m. August 29, 2010

Can anyone take me to a doctor's appointment in San Bernardino on Thursday at 9:30 a.m.? I may end up back in the emergency room, as I am still not myself. I don't know how long this will take. I can always see if someone can take me and someone else can pick me up. Thank you for the prayers and support, I really appreciate it.
>FB Status 4:48 p.m. August 31, 2010

Journal Entry #35:
I am feeling so bad. I have never wanted to go to a hospital so badly in my life. I feel like I am going to die. I don't know how I am going to get help. I will do just about anything at this point.

Thank you for everyone that has been praying for me. Today I feel much better. I will see the doctor tomorrow and find out exactly how I am.
>FB Status 10:37 p.m. September 1, 2010

Being admitted to the hospital for 1 to 5 days.
>FB Status 10:36 a.m. September 2, 2010

Potassium level is 2.5. No wonder I feel yuckie.
            FB Status 1:11 p.m. September 2, 2010

Tomorrow they want to put a tube down my esophagus. I am getting potassium by IV almost nonstop. At midnight they will do another blood test to see how my levels are. I miss my kids.
            FB Status 10:10 p.m. September 2, 2010

Had endoscopy they found some problems. Potassium is up to 3 so far. They want it up to three, five or four. I could go home tonight.
            FB Status 11:43 a.m. September 3, 2010

Omg I just reached 4.0 potassium level. They are working on my magnesium level now. Good chance I can leave tomorrow.
            FB Status 7:31 p.m. September 3, 2010

Potassium went down to 3.7 in the middle of the night. They started supplementing all night again. Please pray that I can get out of the hospital today. I need to be there for Miranda tomorrow.
            FB Status 7:10 a.m. September 4, 2010

Numbers went down again to 3.5 and that's on a potassium drip. Please pray my body can regulate my potassium.
            FB Status 7:51 a.m. September 4, 2010

Normal blood sugar levels, Sleep apnea, Corrected. May be here for a while. Also my microphone on cell phone isn't working. Can only text now.
            FB Status 10:25 a.m. September 4, 2010

Great news. Potassium is up to 4.4. I am waiting to convince a doctor to let me go and to try and get hold of a ride to get me home.

FB Status 6:27 p.m. September 4, 2010

I'm home. Yah!!!! Thank you for all your encouragement. God thank you for keeping me alive.

FB Status 12:31 a.m. September 5, 2010

Check out my new photo, I am healthy. I am so glad.

FB Status 11:34 p.m. September 5, 2010

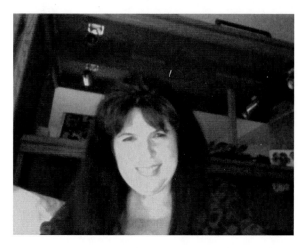

I know you just read many different posts of my Facebook pages. I wanted you to see the sequence of events that transpired to bring me back to health. What happened is all still a blur to me. It's really interesting to look back and see the decline in my health those last few weeks. One minute you feel just fine, and then the slow decline quickly catches up with you and next thing you know you are in the hospital.

As you can see health problems can continue, depending upon the person. Others heal from the surgery, lose weight and don't look back. There are no guarantees in this game. You may wonder if I was thinking to myself that I shouldn't have done the surgery. I continue to say and feel that I would have done it over again a thousand times because I truly believe without that surgery I wouldn't be where I am now.

Anyway at that point, I had just gotten out of the hospital; I was in there for a total of three days. I basically kind of forced my way out. They would have kept me for another day or half day. However, there was something important that I didn't want to miss the next day. I was concerned that if I didn't get home, I wouldn't be there for my daughter's graduation ceremony.

I had Hypokalemia, which is low potassium. I also had low magnesium. Further, the doctor did an endoscopy on me and found loose staples in my stomach. As usual, nothing wanted to stay in me; just like with the sutures that came out. The doctor took the loose staples out of my stomach and now I am able to eat much better. I hadn't felt that good since having the surgery.

The consequence of this procedure was that my appetite increased, and my ability to digest food became easier. That created a new fear in me. I began to fear that all this weight loss success would reverse itself. That was something I had to process through. I did gain weight; I think about ten pounds in the hospital. Because they were pushing those fluids through my system for days, I was bound to gain weight. However, that was good weight. That was really only liquids that after a week or so leveled themselves out. Please be sure to follow your doctor's advice for your dietary needs. It is sometimes difficult for a bypass patient to maintain their nutritional needs, which is why we have specialized supplements to help to that end. Again, as I am not a nutritionist, I will leave that to your doctor to explain your needs and their recommendations for you.

I went through quite a process after I got out of the hospital. I never felt so alone in my life. After all, my children couldn't come to see me, they are just kids. Thank God their father picked them up and took care of them while I was in the hospital. But, other than the wonderful people that helped me to get back and forth to and from the hospital, and watched my house while I was gone, I felt completely alone. Yes, I talked to friends via the phone, but no one came to see me. It really hurt. I began to reevaluate whether I had friends and what changes I needed to make in my life to value myself more, i.e. greater self-care. I won't go into details about the conclusions that I came to, but I just knew that I never wanted an experience like that again. So, I began to formulate a new plan for me. I knew that I needed to feel like I wasn't alone. I have so many friends, they tell me they love me, but why was I so alone at times like these? I have since learned a lot based on this series of events. I believe that was growth on my part and an important shift in my life.

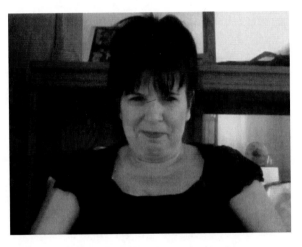

Thank you to everyone, who kicked me in the butt, to help me to get healthy. I know I can be a pain in the butt. I appreciate your love.

FB Status 8:22 p.m. September 15, 2010

I want to be sure to help you understand that there are times when friends and family can't be there for us. People have lives. They are supposed to. I think I set my life up in such a way to think of myself as a victim. I realized that showing up that way in life gave me some positive rewards. It's difficult to think of it that way. However, we don't do anything if we don't receive something from it. Even being a victim has its own rewards. There can be rewards like attention, or people requiring little from you in life, or you requiring little from yourself and so on and so on. I no longer wanted to show up as a victim. This is where that shift happened.

Journal Entry #36:

I don't know what to say. I feel like a new person since I got out of the hospital. I have energy and I have a new clarity and focus like I have never had in my life. I know what my purpose is. To help people that have gone through what I have. People that have been marginalized in society, or been treated as if they were invisible, stupid, lazy or even hard of hearing.. I want to encourage people like me that have been through so much in their lives. I can't wait to start on this new life.

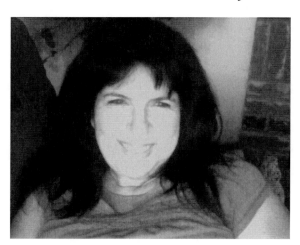

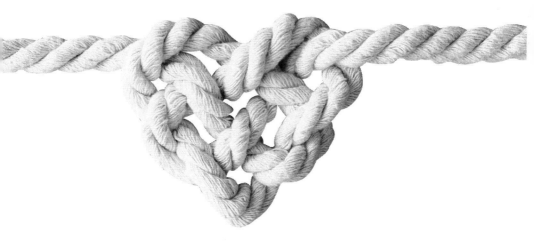

CHAPTER SEVEN

The Magnificent Life

Things began changing at this time. For my son's birthday we went to the fair. I had been out of the hospital only a few days and I was able to walk from early in the day until late in the evening. It's amazing how good you can feel when you have the correct metabolic balance. Today I am wearing size six pants and small sizes in my shirts. My sizes seem to change so rapidly, I can barely keep up. That is huge for me; to like a picture that I am a part of. We liked it enough to but it as a memento of the day. I don't remember a time that I ever looked forward to seeing myself in a photo. Is this part of the new me, not afraid to see myself as other's do? Does this mean I won't be invisible? Can I handle what comes with that? These are all questions that I am pondering and processing through. I wonder when the process ends.

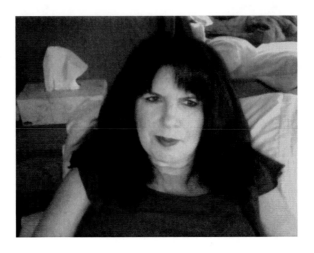

This reminded me of the reason that the doctor's office assessed me with a psychological evaluation before my surgery. I know it must have been a way to weed out those that would be good candidates for the surgery and those that wouldn't. The assessment is important for you and the psychologist to understand if you are ready to do what it takes after you have the surgery. Yes folks, you can actually gain back the weight if your emotional state is not prepared for the changes that will ensue. That's why many doctors require you to diet and show your desire and ability to lose weight before performing the surgery on you. Also there are many emotional reasons why we eat. Without understanding the whys and the hows of the weight gain in the first place, it's possible to gain the weight back. As a therapist, I help clients to process through their emotional baggage and to help motivate them for permanent change. There is an old joke, how many therapists does it take to change a light bulb? The answer is just one, but the light bulb has to want to change. It's the same with this situation. Unless you really want to change, the therapist can't help you to process through the reason for gaining the weight in the first place.

Anyway, at this point, I knew I needed to get a job. It was time. I had the energy, I was healed from my car accidents and it was time to believe that I had value as the therapist I was trained to be. I wanted to work. I needed to work to provide for my kids. I am awake, I am alive, and I am ready to start this new life.

My life soon became filled with memories that I didn't have the energy for earlier. For instance, a few weeks later I took my boys to the beach early in the morning and bought a fresh crab and a fresh shrimp. I didn't know what to do with them; I had never cooked fresh shellfish. I certainly never cooked anything fresh from the sea, or woke up early to drive down to the beach to pick up a live, moving crab and put it in a cooler. I brought the food home, cooked both the crab and one shrimp they had left. I ended up ruining them both. I guess it wasn't about the eating process. It was about a great memory for my children and me.

As I began to feel better, I realized needed a life with people, other than children. In other words, I needed to speak to adults. I began to plan for how to get a new life. I started volunteering my time to feed people at the park. I wanted to make a difference in others' lives. Each week I went to the park. I love chopping up vegetables, so I brought an onion each week and chopped it up to help flavor the food that we were serving; usually hot dogs and hamburgers.

As I reached four months after my surgery, my hair actually did begin to fall out like crazy. I have never seen anything like that. It fell out so much that I actually had a dream that I was going bald. Me, the person who has enough hair for three people on my head usually, I was scared I was going to go bald. Thank God I went to my hairdresser and told her what was happening. She told me that she had some shampoo that helps with hair loss. I started using it and right away and I noticed a difference within a week or two, the hair loss stopped. I wonder when the hair will all come back.

As I continued in this process, I had my ups and downs. Again, I hit a plateau at four months; at least with those numbers on the scale. I knew I must have still been losing inches because my sizes continued to go down. I find myself able to think clearer, focus better, and I am following through more with my own personal paperwork better than I have been able to in years.

Believe it or not, the plumbing is going to get done because the bathroom downstairs started leaking today. How many leaks can a house have? I am beginning to formulate the idea that I want to write a book. When I began journaling this process, I didn't imagine that a book was where this would go. I never felt that I had the ability to be of value. As my self-esteem grows, I realize that I have been limiting myself, working hard to keep myself small and invisible throughout my life. Now I want to make a difference. I encourage you to know that you can make it through this process. Let me help you to understand that you can overcome your emotional obstacles and live the magnificent life. It's only you that has ever stopped you in the first place, and it's only you that can believe in yourself to lie out the life you are intended to live out. That's what I discovered about myself and I began to work toward whatever that magnificent life would turn out to be.

I am beginning to realize that I need to exercise because I am starting to see my skin's elasticity failing me. Especially my arms, they don't look good. I was watching TV the other day. I was watching "the biggest loser". The biggest loser's mom had died and she never saw him lose 219 pounds. I started crying because I realized that my entire life all my mom wanted was for me to lose the weight (I know because she asked me about my weight pretty much any time I talked to her on the telephone and/or saw her in person.) She never got to see me lose the weight. She didn't even know that we looked alike and neither did I. I always said I looked nothing like my mother. I never even knew that I looked just like her until I lost the weight. Now I see my mom in the mirror all the time, and I never thought I looked anything like her. It was all hidden under the layers of fat. I wish she could see me now.

> *Awesome day at church. Planning trunk or treat for Oct. 31st. My job, to pray for others, how great is that. I am in the new season of my life, geez I have only waited for ten years. It feels soooooo good. I can't wait to see what God has in store for me; of course he has only begun to tell me what it all means.*
>
> FB Status 4:03 p.m. October 17, 2010

Journal Entry #37:
I started working on my book and I am getting a billion ideas and I am writing them on bunches of paper. Getting lots done around the house. Starting to think about looking for a job. I have talked to a few people that might prepare letters of recommendations so that I can get a job. I have so many ideas, I just can't get it out of my mind.

Journal Entry #38:
I went shopping with my daughter yesterday…

One interesting part to this process was the fact that my teenage daughter was really struggling with me having this procedure done. Yes, she was a teenager and that has its own difficulties, but this was an unexpected one. It turned out that she was nervous that I would be her size. I laughed when she told me that. I wasn't laughing at her, I was laughing at the concept that I could ever be a size 0 or a size 1. I figured if I made it to size six that would be beyond anything I could imagine. However, this day she and I went shopping at the store. We were in dressing rooms side by side and giving each other things we had brought in to try on. In other words, we were wearing the same size, at least in some shirts. So in a way, what she had been worried about was happening, and it turned out that instead of being upset, she was proud of her mother and what she had accomplished.

Journal Entry #39:

I went to a support group last night and talked to the psychologist about my plan for the book; he was very encouraging to me. We talked about how there are so few books out there about this subject. I told him I plan for the book to be a funny and a serious take on the first year in the life of a gastric bypass patient as said by a therapist that has been through the process herself. I am becoming really serious about this now. I began to write one of the chapters last night and now I want to document daily about my feelings from this point on as well as share the videos I have been filming documenting my weight loss.

Journal Entry #40:

Yesterday was a crazy day. I went to San Diego with a friend who needed to go to a doctor. The car broke down along the way on the side of the freeway. Her husband decided to try and move the car from the traffic on the freeway to help us. Instead, he hurt his calf muscle, I think, or sprained his foot. We took his car to get my friend to her doctor's appointment. He had the car towed nearby and the tow truck driver drove him to the emergency room. We went to her doctor's appointment then we picked up her husband on the way home. After all that, I found out none of my three kids took their house key with them to school, so they had to sit outside on our lawn for an hour waiting for me to come home after that entire adventure. What an interesting life I have, never a dull moment.

OMG - I just bought size 4 pants. I'm still in shock.
FB Status 4:53 p.m. October 24, 2010

Journal Entry #41:

I am super hungry today and then I had my first difficult blood sugar attack. I think I ate too much fruit and carbs today that set the blood sugar attack off. After that happened, I made a decision to quit eating crackers. I won't be buying them anymore. I have been so hungry these last two days. Should I have hunger so soon after surgery? Is eating the carbs causing the problems? I think I need to get back on the two protein shakes per day diet and exercise.

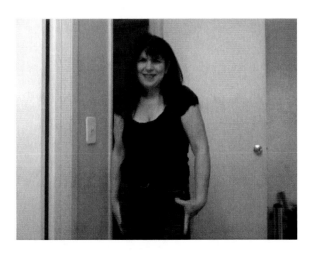

Journal Entry #42:

Well it was bound to happen I suppose, I was asked out on a date today. I just told my daughter and she is really, really upset with me. I didn't think that would be a problem because she had previously assured me that she would not have any issues with me dating, but she clearly does. I rarely was asked out on dates before the surgery. Ok, so I need to tell you about my first date. It was bad, did I say bad? He spent the entire time talking about himself, his ex-girlfriend, and his ex-wife. Granted, I am a therapist-type person, so I asked him about his life. I didn't know that he would hijack the conversation. He never got off the subject of how he has no money (while he is taking me out on a date). It was like he was trying to make me feel guilty so I would pay. Seriously? Anyway, then I told him I couldn't eat any sweets so he takes me out to Starbucks and orders himself a muffin or something and I can't eat or drink anything there. After that I was so hungry I just told him to take me home. Well, I guess I had to get the first date out of my system. But seriously, did it have to go so badly?

Journal Entry #43:
I went to church today. Then a friend wanted to go by our old church and see some old friends. I thought it sounded fun. Quickly, I realized that I didn't belong on this trip. First of all, people I have known for years didn't recognize me. It was as if I didn't even exist, I felt completely invisible. I was able to connect with one girl that was thinking about doing the lap band. Other than that, I learned that this was a weird feeling. Do I tell the person who I am when they don't recognize me? Am I trying to elicit compliments when I do that? It feels like that, so I don't want to tell them who I am. The whole thing just felt weird.

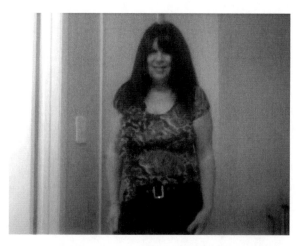

Now yesterday I went to another old church and had that same feeling that I didn't exist. I ran into about four or five people

that I knew, one didn't really recognize me and some of the other people did. Those times I received genuine compliments and really enjoyed catching up with the person just to catch up. I think I will stay away from some of these places for a while. I did make a point of saying hi to someone who was working in the classroom, but she looked at me and didn't know who I was. She was busy in the classroom, so I left it at that. I couldn't get out of there quick enough. I know that I am on a journey and right now part of this process is bringing balance to who I am in my head and who I really am, both physically and mentally.

This will become a theme for me for years to come. Reintroducing myself to people I have known for years, reminding them of how I knew them and when I knew them. Even being asked to provide a picture of myself before the surgery so that they can remember our relationship, was all a part of the process.

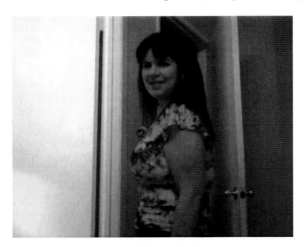

Journal Entry #44:
Today was the first Thanksgiving that I didn't have my kids, and also the first one since my surgery. I was invited to a few different places. I didn't feel good. I was up two nights with stomach problems. When I woke up today, I had lost my first

pound in over two weeks. Anyway, I was afraid I wouldn't be able to eat. I was getting sick all the way up until the moment that I went to my friend's house. I did fine when I got there. I picked out a few things to eat. I brought a salad of cranberries and walnuts. I had a little of that, although I was afraid to use the salad dressing that I had brought. It might be too much sugar for my system. I had a little ham, turkey, and asparagus with a small portion of mashed potatoes and acorn squash. They had put in brown sugar and then asked if I could have it. I told them I'm not sure, but not to worry about me. After all, I can take care of my food needs just fine. I wore my smallest size four pants and a size small shirt. I did fine, food-wise. In fact, I am trying to be very careful that I don't gain weight between Halloween, Thanksgiving, Christmas, and New Years. Thus far, I am still losing weight and not gaining it. That is good news, especially for the holidays.

I'm still struggling in so many areas. I know that this sounds depressing, but I want to be real with all of my feelings, as some of you may be experiencing these thoughts and are wondering if it is normal or not. When you see old friends when they knew you as someone else...it tends to bring on the old feelings you used to have during that time in your life. Like if they knew you as a nerd then when they see you again, you are still a nerd to them (when in fact you are Miss Popular). It definitely brings out old low self-esteem stuff and I just don't want to be someone who acts like I am all that because I lost weight. The other thing I am experiencing is a little weird. When you get this small, you may have to shop in the junior section to get some things to fit. That may sound cool, but it is kind of weird and embarrassing at the same time. It's like you begin to feel younger and smaller. It's hard to know who you are. It's all a part of some of the emotional issues that you may experience through this process. Everyone is different and every experience is different, try not to judge yourself during your process.

Journal Entry #45:

It's November 26th and I have lost one pound in almost the last three weeks. I was thinking that that was all I lost this month but then I looked back and I am still on track for 5-6 pounds every month. It's so easy to think you are getting nowhere in this process without looking back to see your successes. I still eat a good amount. I can eat two tacos in a sitting. It used to be eight, seven, or six. At least now I only have two. Yeah, I am definitely going through a lot of changes. I think I look older now. I didn't used to look this old. I think this is a side effect from the surgery. I'm thinking as time passes my skin's elasticity will bounce back.[19]

I decided I'm going to start dating, or at least to being receptive to the idea. Wow, this is a big deal. To think that I could trust in the dating process is a big step for me. I struggled with this idea for many years for several reasons. I didn't want my daughter to think that you need a man. Conversely, I think I taught her she didn't need a man. Also, she was struggling with the concept of me dating and I didn't want to upset her. I had been alone for so long. Since she was my oldest, I was uncertain how this would impact her. Even though I am alone on holidays, I have great friends and I am not feeling lonely in that way. But, I know I am not pushing forward with my life and I feel that it is time to do that.

Homemade tomatillo salsa, came out awesome. Oven fried potatoes with great seasoning. Homemade pizza, ok I didn't make the dough, however the rest was shear genius. In case you were wondering, I cooked all day, so the above named dishes were not served together.

FB Status 7:52 p.m. November 27, 2010

Today I played volleyball for the first time in years. I was definitely rusty at my game, but the totally awesome news, I was able to set with no pain. I couldn't take the smile off of my face, for anyone who knows me, you know my love of the game, and to be able to play again was sheer heaven.

FB Status 1:05 a.m. November 30, 2010

I was just thinking how interesting it is that each bariatric surgeon seems to have different recommendations for their patients before and after surgery. One of the more interesting things to me is that my doctor prescribes potassium for three months after the surgery. However, I almost died because I didn't take my potassium. So, shouldn't that mean that all doctors should prescribe this? Also, some doctors allow you to eat what you want right away. They tell you to introduce the foods slowly, one at a time, as you are adding to your diet. My doctor recommends that we eat no carbohydrates for the first 75% of our weight loss. He knows that we have a small window in which to lose weight. He just wants us to get it done. I wonder if there will be some guidelines that are followed across the board with bariatric surgeons as they continue to learn what works and doesn't work with their patients.

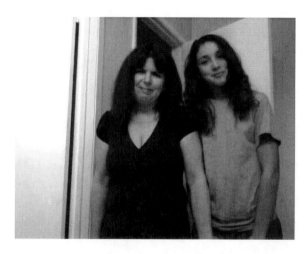

Journal Entry #46:
Played volleyball for the first time in many years. I didn't feel curtailed by my weight. I could breathe well. My ability to move much faster was amazing. Plus of course, you couldn't peel the smile off of my face as anyone who knows me knows what volleyball means to me. I ran into a girl that I played with years before. She didn't comment on my weight, although I could tell she saw the difference. We were on the same team, so we had to sit out together while another team came on the court. We were talking about how I had left the church about a year before, and I visited them on Sunday morning not too long ago and people I had known for years didn't recognize me. I told her how uncomfortable that felt. Also, how so many people that I knew had left the church and there were so many new people there now. She mentioned that she had lost about 85-90 lbs. a year and a half ago and the same thing happened to her. She exercised real hard to lose the weight and then got stuck and eventually went back to overeating and gained it all back plus five pounds. I asked if the way people treated her differently had affected her and how it did. I asked about her identity and how that was different during those times, i.e. she felt invisible as a person who was overweight. She said people don't seem to recognize her in the same way, and then she felt uncomfortable because she had lost weight many times as most of us had, so when she lost weight people didn't acknowledge it and when she gained it back when people saw her coming they didn't want to say anything and lock eyes because it was like "here she comes again and now she has gained the weight back." I felt a deep compassion for her story and I empathized with her. I hope I don't gain this weight back, and I remain a success story. I have been really hungry this week, I didn't expect that for the first year. Of course, I am expecting my cycle again and I have noticed that my hunger does seem to be greater right before that time.

Journal Entry #47:

It is December 3rd, 2010, one more day until my six month anniversary since my surgery. I have lost 87 pounds and my hair did fall out tons, and tons, and tons. Actually, I wish it would stay this way because it's much easier to take care of when it is not as thick. You know, I feel really healthy. Considering dating more, I started responding to some of the online stuff. I guess my newer pictures elicit guys to want to date me, or talk to me or something. However, I am scared, I don't want to be hurt and it's hard to trust men. I want to lose the rest of this weight but I don't know how much more I want to lose. I can't believe the difference in me from six months ago to today. I look at pictures of me, it's like I was so unhealthy and now I just feel so different and I know I'm still not done losing weight. Really happy that I have the energy that I do.

Journal Entry #48:

Went to doctor on December 14th. What an experience. I got my blood test results back. They were really good for the most part. My cholesterol was awesome! My potassium was great! My vitamin levels were good, too! My liver results were still off. They said that takes 18 months to two years to completely respond from the weight loss changes. The only problem that I had was my thyroid, which has never been off. One of the numbers related to my thyroid was high and the other number was low. I had no idea what that meant. So as most people do, I googled the exact numbers on the internet and it seemed like the consensus was that I had hyperthyroidism. Knowing of course that googling is not a useful tool for diagnosis, I made an appointment with my primary doctor. Not bad huh, at least I am handling this part correctly. From what I can tell, I may have to be on thyroid medication. That is scary, what if I stop losing weight, or maybe I am losing so slowly because of the hyperthyroidism, I read that that can happen as well. Yes, I Google way too much. The nurse asked me if I wanted to know what my BMI (Body Mass Index) was when I walked into her office. I said yes, she told me 50%. I was shocked. I had no idea, that it had been so high. Anyway it turns out that now it is 25.6. Which is a few pounds away from a normal percentage. 24.9 would be the high end of normal. I am so very happy about this. She is happy with what I weigh now. I know the doctor wants me to lose a lot more weight; I can't ever imagine that happening. Today I went shopping for the second time this week and I am completely in a size three. I had to start looking at new sizes because I am getting plumbers butt. My pants are falling off of me and showing my little bootie. So, I felt that it was time to see if I am really in other sizes. My only goal has been to probably be a size two, since that is the size that I think I am supposed to be. Judging by my weight and my pant size, I think that it is possible for this to happen. Anyway I am so stoked. It is funny how fat I still look in clothes. Don't imagine that! I would hate to have to pay for your therapy! Anyway, I feel very hungry all the time now, so I am eating a lot. I haven't lost anything in the last week or so, so I am surprised that I had gone down another size. From a size 16 to a three in six months and I am, for the most part, healthy. I am tired at times, having trouble sleeping, and a little moody. But, in comparison to my life before, this surgery has given me a whole new life. This was my dream. However, I never really imagined that it would come true.

I am speaking to the support group meeting on the 27th of January. I have asked my children to be there. I still can't believe the passion that I feel about this subject and what has happened to others and to me, too. I ran into a friend of mine today at Wal-Mart. She just finished her degree to be an R.N. She thinks the complications are being underestimated. I agree with her. The statistics for this surgery seem lower than I believe they actually are, but I am no expert. I would love to see how these statistics are created and what the research data is, etc. She told me every patient said the same thing that I did about being willing to do it again in a heartbeat because we had no life before the surgery and we are blessed beyond measure after the surgery (even with complications). That says a lot for the success of this surgery. I wonder how many people that did the lap band will end up having the gastric bypass. Another thought just to ponder.

Just got a gift from my sons, sugar free gum and sugar free mints in the flavors that I love. It may not seem like a lot, but for me, I have to say that was the perfect gift. I am so happy.

FB Status 4:54 p.m. December 22, 2010

It's My Birthday. Happy Birthday Me!!! This is going to be a great year.

FB Status 9:20 a.m. December 22, 2010

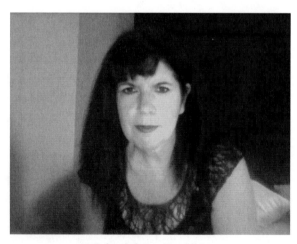

My birthday in Las Vegas
December 25, 2010 Merry Christmas!

Journal Entry #49:

I decided not to post on my Facebook page that I was down to a size three. I don't want to sound like I am egotistical, even though I am in a way. In fact, I don't know that I would ever post about my size again. Even if I were not egotistical, I think it would undeniably make me appear to be. The truth is, when I hit size four, I was so shocked. I had only owned a size four once and it was a pair of pants. To think that my size four pants were getting big and that I needed to go down in size was shocking; but not as shocking as when I initially realized I had hit being a size four. I am kind of sad in a way. Why shouldn't I say that I am a size three out loud? I am too concerned of what people would think about me to yell it from the rooftops. I really only told the closest people in my life, unless someone specifically asked. It has been several weeks since I have lost weight. However, this is the holidays and it is a miracle that I haven't gained any weight during this time. I hope to get back on track after the holidays. I still have 10-20 pounds to go and I need to take advantage of the weight loss window I am in so that I can actually lose some weight during this time.

It's official, as of this morning I have a healthy BMI. OMG 24.9. The sky is the limit now. Watch out world.

                    Facebook 11:57 a.m. January 3, 2011

Journal Entry #50:

It's official, omg! My weight today is 133, my first big goal of this whole process! My BMI is officially 24.9, "healthy." This is all I could think about from day one; to have a healthy BMI seemed to be unreachable, and yet today I am here. My surgery was June 4th, so the seven month anniversary of my surgery is tomorrow, and I have hit a healthy BMI. I am so happy. Actually to be honest, I am now only losing about four pounds a month and it is getting slower all the time. I did sign up to join a boot camp for weight loss. I was hoping to rev up my metabolism and take advantage of this window that could close by the end of the year. I know people lose weight after that, but to me that it is the easiest time in which to still lose weight. So how much more do I want to lose? That is a great question, Carol. I don't know. I'm thinking around 120 should be my goal. Just to imagine that I am starting off 2011 healthy. I would have never thought it was possible.

I have decided to take a seminar called "The One" this Saturday. The purpose of the seminar is to help people be more effective in helping their community. My little park feeding group has already decided to branch out and merge with another group so that we can help more people in more ways. In fact, Wednesday we are meeting to do a mission statement on how we can help the homeless in the Inland Empire more effectively. It seems that right now many get caught up in a viscous cycle. Typically, they get caught for loitering, get ticketed, can't pay the ticket, get a warrant for their arrest, go to jail, get out of jail, and then start the process all over again. We realize this is probably due to there being no where for them to sleep, go to the bathroom, keep warm, shower, or clean and store their clothing. Our country has to step up and do something. With this economy, things are getting worse, not better. This became our new goal; to help identify resources in our community that can help to break that cycle.

Journal Entry #51:
The world is opening up for me, and frankly I am scared. I have never lived up to my potential and calling in my life. Now I feel that it is starting. I am so excited, but I also want to run. I was asked to speak Jan. 27th at this support group and give my testimony, because I am a huge success story. Who would have thunk? But I know it's my calling. I also spoke at my church

this weekend about the weight loss and what I have done since I have felt physically fit. I feel like I am less and less invisible all the time.

I look just like my mother. All my life I never looked like her. Now that I have lost weight, I realized that I always did. I miss her and it is a little weird seeing her in the mirror. I love you Mom.

FB Status 1:25 p.m. January 15, 2011

Journal Entry #52:
Yesterday, I took my daughter shopping since she wanted to spend the money she received for Christmas. I love shopping these days! Anyway, on the way to the store, she started saying to me, "Don't you feel that you took the easy way out?" She had been watching the series "I Used to Be Fat" on TV. She decided since these young kids could lose the weight easily, that I took the easy way out. It took me a minute to be able to formulate a response to her. At first I felt so defensive. It took everything I had to not respond from that place. I tried to help her understand that my health was minimal at best before the surgery. I tried to remind her about our lives before all these changes. I asked her if she thought that physical exercise was the only thing hard about losing weight. I said, "After everything you watched me go through, you really think that I took the easy way out?" I reminded her of my low potassium and what could have happened to me without treatment. I tried to explain to her that even though I had lost 50-70 pounds many times, it just never stayed off and I never, ever reached my goal. I tried to explain to her how slow my metabolism was compared to others.

I got nowhere. Then I realized that if she sees me that way, than I guess that's just how she sees me. How many other family members still secretly in their heart feel that way about the person that has lost the weight? How many other family members resent the person that has lost weight and sometimes doesn't say it? Teenagers often don't have a filter and they say what many others might be thinking. I decided that what she was telling me I needed to hear. It's important to understand what the family member/friend may be feeling and the process they are going through. They are a huge piece of this puzzle. Becoming this new person doesn't happen in a bubble.

I just got a call from my doctor's office to confirm speaking at their weight loss seminar. I was asked to speak for 10-15 minutes. Those meetings are usually packed. I am surprised that it is me that is speaking. She assured me that if I get nervous she will help prompt me with questions to answer. I was nervous; I was thinking ten to fifteen minutes is a lot of time to speak. I pray that I come up with everything that I want to say there. I already have an outline for my talk, but I need to write something down before I get there.

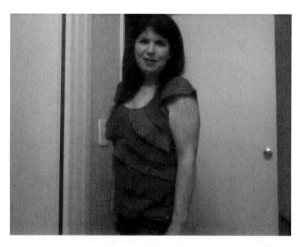

Decided the best way to write the speech was to get caught up on my book and then pull the outline from the book, got about 35 pages of my book tentatively done with another ten pages of

notes that I need to look at and flesh into chapters. Next step make outline for my speech.

> FB Status 8:54 p.m. January 25, 2011

I am ready to write out my index cards. Tomorrow, I practice, practice and go kick butt.

> FB Status 8:16 p.m. January 26, 2011

Index Cards Done, Practice Done, Looking Awesome (In Process) .Almost There!

> FB Status 1:55 p.m. January 27, 2011

Speech went awesome. It was really fun. Check out the pic.

> FB Status 9:14 p.m. January 27, 2011

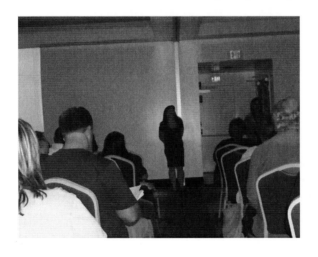

Journal Entry #53:

Last night I spoke at a weight loss seminar for new patients. I felt like this was a turning point in my life. It was a beginning; a new season where I am to help work with and encourage bariatric patients. I prepared a testimony that lasted for fifteen minutes. I have to say I wondered if I was too real when I spoke. I included all the complications and problems that I ran into after my surgery. I also made it completely clear that even with all the worse case scenarios that I hit, I still would do the surgery a million times over again. It was weird to see the last picture the doctor had taken of me pre-surgery, set up behind me. My daughter was tripping out! She had never realized how big I was until she saw that picture. It's amazing how the people around you don't really see it. It's like they become immune to it. I spoke with the psychologist after I spoke and discussed with him my desire to give the friends and family members of bariatric patients a voice. All they say at the meetings is that I am the support person for (enter name). Do we get to hear how they feel? Is there dialogue about their struggles? Do we talk about how the relationships in the patient's life can become strained due to the surgery?

When a patient changes in a system, the system, i.e. family, has to change too. People hate change. They are afraid of it and thus everyone wants to fight to put the system back to where it was. It isn't possible for things to stay the same after the surgery. Everything looks different by design. Where is the place for the friends and family to go and share? I want to do a support group that addresses this issue.

I took a stack of index cards with me when I spoke. I was nervous and I thought this would help me to remember what I had been through and what happened through the weight loss process. These are my note cards from my speech:

Breathe deep while looking down, then breathe, exhale and look up.

Look at the audience, speak slowly.

Name, surgery, date, 224 starting weight.

Life before, high cholesterol.

High Blood pressure, bed ridden, sleep-apnea, c-pap machine.

Back pain, asthma, fibromyalgia.

After surgery, pain, seepage, sutures, hormones flooding.

Water hurt, everything tastes different, ice chips, 24 lbs.

First week.

Can't drink teas, dumping.

Quit taking my meds, no vitamins or c-pap.

No potassium, no exercise, advantages feeling great.

Paperwork, energy, napping, not hungry, 42 lbs.

Watching Food network, cooking, weight loss chart.

Goal setting every 5 pounds and BMI.

One month. Smaller sizes, BMI down 110, buffet child price.

Plateau 8 days, San Diego trip 3 weeks.

Two months 47, denial how did I get so big.

Grieving.

Hormones, dumping, smell like syrup embarrassing.

Ketosis, hamburger, salads, veggies, communion.

Cymbalta overdose nausea, 2½months, wardrobe ½ gone.

Tired, nausea, oak glen, first hospital.
Hands/feet, 2100 potassium, hypokalemia.

Second hospital

3 days potassium, magnesium, dehydration.

Banana bags, fluids, endoscopy, feels great.

Eating more, fair walking, picture Newport Beach 65 lbs.

3.5 mo. sizes 6 and 8 support groups.

Writing book, hair falling out, vitamins?

4 mo. 75 lb. chili, passion.

5 mo. 81 lbs. down, size 3, first date.

Teenager, not recognized, embarrassing, reintroduce myself.

Shorter?, 5 lbs/month Pismo, Las Vegas.

Volleyball, back pain, watermelon/oranges, salsa.

6 mo. 90 lbs. doctor-cholesterol, protein.

Vitamin levels, thyroid, liver, speaking seminar—omg

7 mo. normal BMI 24.9 wow, 5 lbs. month.

Park feeding, Christmas tree lot, involved at church.

Homeless coalition, Fontana Community Coalition

Bible study, my kids, boot camp.

Writing a book—dream, BMI 240, MFT help bariatric patients

91 lbs. 10 to go

Would I do this again? Absolutely

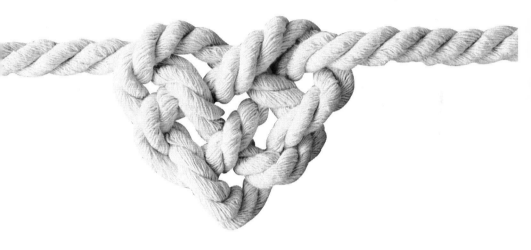

CHAPTER EIGHT

I Met Someone

Life can sure take a turn sometimes.
                    FB Status 10:09 pm February 10, 2011

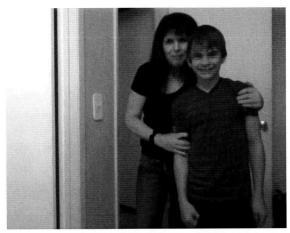

Current picture of me and my 13 year old son Brian.

Well, this is the point in my journal where my life takes a huge turn. This is the one place that I struggled with sharing with readers about. I guess I felt shame and embarrassment and didn't know how to write about my choices from this point forward. As I look back now, this time between finishing my book and publishing my book was necessary. I am actually six and a half years out from my procedure as I write these words.

Let me tell you what happened. I met a guy. Not so shocking to think about, people meet significant others all the time. I was seven months out from my surgery and there he was. No one I could have ever expected to be in my life. On paper, this guy didn't look great. Nonetheless, I fell in love and I felt like my life was going very fast, way too fast for me to handle. I didn't know how to put the brakes on. I guess I can honestly say that I didn't know what it felt like for a man to look at me and see me as beautifully as he saw me and to this day still continues to see me.

It is a little heady to go from being morbidly obese, where I felt marginalized in society, to being the most beautiful girl in the world to one man. I can definitely tell you that that is the way he sees me. He wakes up in the morning telling me that I am beautiful and it is one of the last things that he says to me at night.

However, that being my experience, I did turn the world upside down for myself and my children when he came into our lives. The children were used to having me for themselves, and that changed drastically. They didn't want to accept him. Especially, due to the fact that he had done things in his past that were beyond questionable. I, on the other hand, saw past those things and saw a man that had a heart of gold. You know the cliché that says you don't know him the way I know him? Well, I played that out to the fullest of my being. I wanted to feel beautiful. I wanted a man that could fix those things that were broken in me; to turn my six-foot tall weeds into a beautiful sanctuary in my backyard.

What I didn't account for was that I really wasn't ready for this. This is where I tell you; do as I say not as I do. There is an old saying in 12-step recovery, don't make any decisions for that first year of your recovery. There are many reasons for that. One of them being that you might make a different decision if you took the time and patience to do so. Another reason could be that if you take that time and make that same decision; at least you are making it from a more informed position. So, recognizing that I was in the middle of a roller coaster of emotions, feelings and body changes, it would have been beneficial to wait until I felt ready. This guy was impulsive. I honestly felt that he was afraid that once I finished losing weight that another guy would snatch me up and he would lose his chance to date me. So he pursued and pursued, as Steve Harvey states in his book men are made to pursue, provide and protect.[20] He convinced me he was going to do these things for me in spades.

I will go into more details later in the next couple of chapters. But, in a nutshell, we moved things along extremely fast! I think he told me he loved me in a few days! Ladies, if you are hearing this, keep in mind that it is way too soon to know what you are feeling. He tried to marry me somewhere in that first week. I was able to stop the train and hold him off for an entire two and a half months. My friends and family did almost everything to stop me. However, I didn't listen. I don't think I could even hear a word they were saying at that point. I tried to control things in small ways, like requesting a simple wedding with just the two of us and my kids. Instead, I gave in and it turned into a lovely wedding at a friend's house. It was an inexpensive potluck-type wedding in a lovely backyard. We began our lives with a wonderful honeymoon and life changed from there on in. But like I said, I will get back to that story a little bit later.

It's official—100 pounds as of today. It's time to parteeeeeeee!
FB Status 9:40 a.m. February 12, 2011

Check it out, I am back to life. I have my first job interview tomorrow. I pray that I get experience in the interviewing process and if it is the right job for me that I would get the job.
FB Status 11:02 a.m. February 14, 2011

Talk about a crazy day, I have a job interview, then I meet for the first time with my marriage family therapist supervisor. Then my son has an interview to see if he makes it in ASB at his high school, then my daughter and I have a meeting to sign up for AP classes at the same school. I am very excited and very proud of my children.

FB Status 7:40 a.m. February 15, 2011

Interview went awesome. Lots of fun got along great with the director. At the very least it was a great first time interview experience. Supervision was amazing as well. What a blessing. I am amazed with the way God is working in my life right now. Thank You God.

FB Status 12:38 p.m. February 15, 2011

Is the world spinning, or is just me?

FB Status 6:06 p.m. February 17, 2011

Where do you shop when you get so small? In the junior department, the sizes are odd and in the petite section, the sizes are even. So, I end up going back and forth as I lost weight from the petite section to the junior section since they all carry different types of clothing. There is certainly not professional wear in the junior section. I also started going to stores with my daughter that carry junior clothes because they fit so much better than the other stores. They allow for the maturity of my body and also for my smallness at the same time. What a change from the beginning of the process until now. My head is spinning. I don't feel like I even belong in this life. I was a size 16 to 18 when I started and now at times I can't find things small enough to fit me. I am looking in the mirror and I can't believe what I see.

It is fun to go shopping with my daughter and bring most of the same sizes into the room and swap back and forth what we try on. I couldn't even begin to envision that this was a possibility, but she could. I was losing weight and getting attention because of it. I think she felt threatened that I was intruding into her territory and thus I was going to start acting like a kid and what kid wants her mother to do that? She wouldn't even acknowledge my weight loss for quite some time. Think about it, if I appear to be like a teenager, how does a teenager process those feelings? It couldn't have been easy. Generally, changes aren't easy. The kids loved my ability to function, show up and suit up in their lives, which was something I wasn't able to do before.

My boys had no problem in accepting these changes right away. However, my daughter wanted and/or needed all these changes to go away. To be fair, she just needed a little time and in the end we became closer than ever. In fact to this day, she still "borrows" my clothing quite frequently. Who would have guessed that would happen?

I don't quite understand why she felt threatened by fat, old me and the possibility that I could get smaller. I guess part of it is a teen girl thing. The interesting thing is that at around four or five months after my surgery date, her attitude started completely changing. She got excited to go shopping with me to find clothes that fit me properly. Like she became my shopper, and could treat me like a Barbie doll. I really loved and still do love our time together when we do girly things like clothes shopping, eye brows, manicures, and pedicures. I really didn't care about taking care of my appearance in that way before the surgery. I didn't have the energy and I didn't look good in the clothes. I also think I have gone through this process where I am reliving my teenage years again! Gee, I wonder if that was why my daughter felt threatened. It is almost as if I was growing up and learning how to do things that I skipped during that time in my life. Even though I weighed less throughout my life, I never felt like a girly girl, which now I do more often than not. I like to dress up and look pretty and that is a weird shift from the old woman that I felt like I was right before the surgery. Not having the energy to go to Los Angeles and have some fun for the day (like when we went to La Brea Tar pits and I fell asleep while everyone was having fun and someone snapped a picture of what I now call my "beached whale pic."). It's funny that that picture is now my badge of courage. Eventually, we went back to that same location and tried to duplicate that picture. What I didn't realize was that it was an impossible feat to perform. We took many pictures with the same positioning, but no picture could live up to the original.

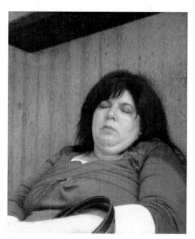 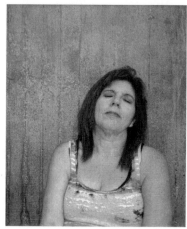

Journal Entry #54:

It is February 24, 2011 and I reached my goal of size 2 a few days ago! Couldn't get by the fact that my size 3's were falling off my butt! My new pants have room in them so I believe that I will be making it to size 1 before long. I am humbled and amazed at all the differences in my body. Someone came up to me the other day at church. She was checking out the website for the church and saw some pictures from Easter. It has been 8 ½ months since my surgery. How can so many things change so quickly? She was saying to me how I must have been going through so much psychologically when my body was changing so fast. I told her that I am continually working through my feelings in that regard. Oh how many things have changed.

I am dating someone now that I love and I don't think that would have happened without the weight loss. I am moving closer to that first job as a therapist intern. I am going to a seminar tomorrow to work on some new areas in my life. It has been 8½ months since my surgery, how can so many things change so quickly.

Alright I am going to say it, I'm in love and I don't care who knows!

FB Status 10:41 a.m. March 3, 2011

I played volleyball at church last night. It feels so good to have a body that listens to me and allows me to have an awesome time.

FB Status 6:46 a.m. April 4, 2011

Journal Entry #55:

Its April 20, 2011, my daughter turned 16 yesterday! I can't believe that I have a child that is 16 years old. I am in the process of planning my wedding and so much has happened these last 3½months. My weight remains the same and has for nearly two months. I would like to lose five more pounds to reach my goal. Five pounds, that is nothing, and not extremely important anymore. I am virtually the person that I hope to remain, and/ or within a few pounds here or there. It is becoming clearer that this new me, is me, both physically and emotionally. The surgery did exactly what it was intended to do. It gave me back my life, or maybe it gave me my life for the first time.

A good third of my hair fell out, it's starting to come back in my hairdresser said, it's going to come back in, it's just taking time.[21]

As I may have mentioned before, throughout this first year I continued to attend support groups with other weight loss patients. Those groups were so helpful and so informative in learning about nutrition, understanding the ways in which our body changes through this process, and the psychological feelings that we all go through. To be able to process these feelings in a group setting was so effective for me. I was sad to hear that a majority of patients tend to not attend these types of meetings. They were missing out. I made friendships that still play a role in my life today.

At this stage, I still don't eat sugar, drink soda or alcohol. I made a decision to not go down that slippery slope of weight gain again. My understandings of the statistics are that patients, on average, regain 40% of their weight loss at some point. I definitely do not want to fit into those statistics. In fact, sitting here many years later, I can honestly say I am pretty happy with my weight. Yes, I could stand to lose about ten pounds, but that is a far cry from needing to lose a hundred pounds.

Journal Entry #56:
It's April 30th. I've been so happy about a decision I have made in my life. It has changed everything! I'm getting married to a gorgeous man with a good heart and is good to my kids. Would this man have come into my life otherwise? Good question. When I ask him that question, he always says he would have seen my heart and not my weight, but I don't think that's true.

Later on, at a support group, he was able to see a huge picture of me that we taken just before my surgery date. In a weak moment, he said he wasn't sure if he would have seen me when I was overweight. I know that all of you ponder these kinds of thoughts. If you are married already and have the procedure, you go through your own special process that we will discuss later on. If you aren't in a relationship, you begin to see that your choices become less limited. My husband once told me that he heard there was a study done, that concluded attractive people were hired and made more money than less attractive people.[23] Isn't that sad and interesting at the same time? It's an interesting fact, but sad that it is true. It turned out that as I lost the weight I continued to make more money and be more successful. This tells you that you, too, could make more money and have more success in your life. I guess we live in a fairly shallow world.

Expect to have your feelings possibly go up and down during the process of understanding the new you and accepting that you have the ability to do more now than you have ever done before. Both in your career and in your personal life, changes will happen. It is freeing and a bit heady, but that is something that you will need to process through during this first year or two. I have to admit that I didn't want my man to see my old pictures. I wanted him to only see me as I am now. Again, as I sit here many years later, I have come to terms with being proud of what I have accomplished and realizing there is nothing to be embarrassed about any more.

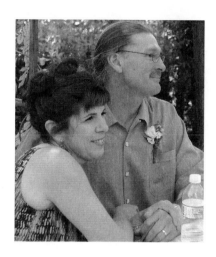

Journal Entry #57:

It's April 30, 2011. I got married today. Who would have thought that would happen? Of course, I moved too fast. I think this is a product of the weight loss surgery and maybe a husband who is a bit impulsive. The theme of the wedding is the ocean. My dress is blue, his shirt is blue with flip flops, and my children all have clothing in a shade of blue; casual beach attire. The garden and pond at my friend's house are beautiful. I still can't believe that she did all this for us. The wedding was simple, and the wind didn't turn out to be a problem at all. We ended up being married by the Captain of a ship, which was something important to my husband. I never could have imagined all those pounds ago that I would be getting married within the year. There were approximately fifty people in attendance, including those people that suggested we wait. They still supported us, because they loved us. All in all, it was a special day.

We went on a honeymoon in San Clemente. My husband suggested trying some wine. I didn't drink wine before my surgery. Now I know it is getting close to my first year, but I never thought of drinking wine. I have been very careful about drinking all these years for many reasons. The first of which is that I don't like wine. Wine gives me headaches. Secondly, I have children and I don't want to model bad behavior for them. I have spoken to many people post-surgery and watched them chose to drink alcohol or not to drink alcohol. I know that post-surgery alcohol affects us greater.[24] What if I had an adverse reaction? I had heard stories from people at the support group stating they got really sick after drinking alcohol and wouldn't do it again. Plus, there are the concerns about finding a new drug of choice. Food was my addiction. It is so easy to chose a new drug of choice and remain in denial about that new choice being a problem. I did drink a sip of alcohol and I didn't die. But I plan on taking a "watch and see" attitude about any alcohol use in the future. After all, aren't there calories in alcohol?

I am able to eat foods that I couldn't have before. I tried a cupcake after my wedding. I made cupcakes as part of the dessert for the reception. Anyway, I was able to have a cupcake and a small amount of frosting. My stomach reacted a little; it felt a little bubbly. I was ok, though. What am I doing? I have so many friends that at some point eat things with sugar after their surgery. I keep thinking that if they can do it, then I can do it, too. As long as it is in moderation right? In the back of my head, I am wondering if this is going to bite me in the butt.

On honeymoon day five. San Clemente is gorgeous.
                    FB Status 7:12 p.m. May 5, 2011

Journal Entry #58:
On the way back from my honeymoon in San Clemente. Wow! Just had the most amazing time! So beautiful and I never dreamed that life could be like this! Hit my 11 month anniversary while we were there and have been married for a few days. Without the surgery none of this was possible, none of it. At least that is what I told myself.

Journal Entry #59:

May 10th, 2011. Today I went to go get the mail. Our mailbox is across the street from the house. As I came back, I saw my neighbor outside. He looked at me and talked to me for the first time in about a year. All of a sudden, his eyes grew wide, and then wider and then he said, "Carol?" I'm like, yeah it's me. He said, "Wow, you look really good." I said, "thank you". He said that all this time he thought someone else had been staying at my house taking care of the kids, when it was me the whole time. You know, I have had so many people not recognize me during this year. People I have known for years and years, but I have to say this one was shocking to me. I guess he really thought I was a different person all this time. I do feel like a totally different person, though. I guess that people have to adjust to my changes just as much as I do.

Journal Entry #60:

May 13, 2011. Well, I have to admit I am beginning to have way too may blood sugar attacks, i.e., hypoglycemia (low blood sugar). I know I am doing something wrong with my diet. I have to get it under control. I have decided to contact the nurse from my doctor's office. I need help in knowing how to stop these problems. It seems like every few days my blood sugar dives and I am asking the kids to get me oranges to get my blood sugar back up. I feel like I am eating to get my blood sugar up way too many times. I know that it is causing my weight to plateau because of needing to balance my blood sugar level. I know that after having surgery sometimes hypoglycemia can become a problem. I already had that problem before my surgery and lately it is out of control.

I am not a medical expert, so I am unable to speak to the medical issues that I was dealing with. All I can say is that if you suspect you are struggling with any of these problems, make an appointment with your doctor. Don't hesitate! Learn about how your body metabolizes sugar and carbohydrates.

Well, I certainly have not been eating this way for a while.

I have been giving myself permission to eat potato chips and salsa, and the salsa has a lot of fruit in it. I like mango salsa, but it doesn't like me. Plus, all the crackers I have had. I gave those up about two weeks ago. It is so weird; crackers were never a problem with me before. Now, they are a huge craving for me. At this point, I have chosen to eat food that is not processed. That makes a difference for me. I enjoy fish, protein, and vegetables.

Journal Entry #61:

I went to my support group tonight, and learned about food marketing techniques. This was very interesting, understanding food labels and how they applied to us, the bariatric surgery patients.

I learned some new things at the support group and made a decision to stop eating crackers. They were a slippery slope to gaining weight. It was up to me to let go of yet another habit that wasn't helping me toward my goal. I ate my first cracker right after I was hospitalized the second time. Something I almost never did pre-op, and then I just began to give myself permission to eat them. First, it was two or three crackers. Then, it became a whole sleeve of them at once. I had gained maybe four pounds and since I stayed within that four-pound range, I didn't really worry about the situation. What I didn't realize, was that I lost nothing else for a long period of time after that. Of course, everyone is telling me how great I look and how I shouldn't lose any more weight. So, I started believing the press, so to speak. What these well-meaning people didn't understand was that although I was small, I still wasn't small enough. You can see in my pictures that many areas of my body still remained bigger than others.

One-year anniversary of my surgery is Saturday. I have now lost 105 pounds. I still have anywhere from one to sixteen pounds to go. Before you say anything, this is not my own personal goal for my body; it was my doctor's idea. I am happy with how I look; I never even dreamt I would be this size.

FB Status June 1, 2011

I visited my doctor and my appointment went really good. One doctor said I could quit losing weight right now, although I will likely gain some weight back in the future, as that is real common. One of the other doctor's wants me to lose 15 more pounds. Then, if I gain a little back, I will be fine.

"Authenticity is a collection of choices that we have to make every day. It's about the choice to show up and be real.
The choice to be honest. The choice to let our true selves be seen."
— **Brené Brown**

The Gifts of Imperfection: Let Go of Who You Think You're
Supposed to Be and Embrace Who You Are

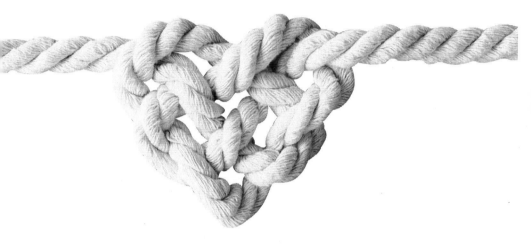

CHAPTER NINE

The Second Year

Journal Entry #62:

It's June 24, 2011. I went to my support group meeting last night. I think this is an important thing to do, guys. They passed out index cards for everyone there. The meeting was packed, so there must have been at least 40 people in the room. The index cards had pictures of different foods and drinks on them. Then we played, "good food" or "bad food". For instance, someone read the card that said, "Chocolate". Everyone screamed "bad". However, if it's dark chocolate, it could be good in limited quantities. Then, someone had the card for sushi. Everyone was unsure. Fish sounds good. However, we all know rice is bad for you. So the answer was bad, sashimi "good". Next, we saw a picture of spaghetti squash, sounds good. However, my doctor suggests that we keep carbs to a minimum before we lose 75% of our weight loss. So, the answer is "bad" before 75% weight loss and "good" after. Well, you get the idea of the game. It was fun and I learned a few things during that game.

We also had a rep from the company that makes some of the surgical instruments the doctor uses in our surgeries. She came to teach us about a computer program that tracks our weight loss, which then communicates with the doctor's office via email to let them know if we are gaining weight and/or on a plateau. The program was quite extensive and something I may avail myself of.

Near the end of the group, three ladies were introduced to the room. They wanted to give a gift to a few people and the gift was a makeover. These three were hairdressers. They all had a heart to help those that lose their hair. One of the hairdressers had cancer and had beaten it many times. So, she wanted to help us through the same process of experiencing hair loss. Wow, everyone said. They want the changes from our body to match with our image in our head. So they were going to give a few people this gift and have a revealing for the changed people at the next support group meeting. I leaned into my daughter, who came to the meeting with me and asked her if she thought I should volunteer myself. As they were taking volunteers, they mentioned they wanted you to be open to any change. I don't remember my daughter's answer. However, I do remember that I decided not to do it. I wasn't sure that I would be open to just anything being done to my hair.

They talked some more about how they wanted to help us because they knew of the hair loss that we went through and how it affected us and our body image. I had lost at least a third of my hair and the hair that was growing back in underneath was a mess. Anyway, I decided not to volunteer and went to go talk to the psychologist that had done my psychological evaluation. I wanted to tell him about my new job and ask how his research for his Ph.D. was coming along. I also wanted to discuss my idea of a support group meeting for the friends/family members of the gastric bypass patients. To make a long story short, ok, I know too late, I was talking to him and out of nowhere one of the girls from the doctor's office grabbed me. We had developed a relationship of sorts when I went into the hospital the second time and she had just changed positions with the doctor. I was the first person that she wheeled into the hospital from the doctor's office because they had to be re-hospitalized. I know, kind of silly. So, now she calls me her "first". She introduces me to her friend, Charisse, the hairdresser, as her "first". Something which I had to explain later, kind of sounded bad if you know what I mean. It turns out that this girl was the catalyst for bringing these three hairdressers to the meeting in the first place. She told me she wanted me to have the makeover. "You have had so many changes and you are in the prime time to begin completely anew." She didn't want me to be mad at her for suggesting me. Deep inside I was thinking, maybe I look terrible and she wanted to help me. I also thought that was so incredibly nice for her to think of me. I really just wanted to sneak out of there so I could remain invisible. After all, I am just one of thousands of patients she had met at the doctor's office. Well, her friend wants to give me a makeover. Will I be open to what she wants to do? I am instantly scared. I like long hair, although I would love a change. I'm always up for a new color on my hair, too. One of my concerns that I shared with her was that I need to be able to put my hair up at night because it bugs me when I sleep. She wants to cut it to my shoulders. Oh yeah, I forgot to tell you, at the beginning of the meeting my daughter leaned into me and said, "Mom, you should cut your hair. It would look so good to your shoulders." At the time, we had no idea the hairdressers were coming to the meeting. I found that to be a confirmation of what Charisse, the hairdresser, wanted to do for me. I told her I was already planning on going to my hairdresser, since my roots were showing. She understood and said we would do this makeover in two stages. The first would be to color the roots and possibly a cut and the second would be closer to the next meeting on July 28th, when we would make all the final changes. So in that order, we will do haircut, color and highlights. I thought to myself highlights, I never had that done. I do the bare minimum to get by. I had been planning on doing a photo shoot, sounds big, but I just meant go to Sears or somewhere and get some one-year pics for the book. So I guess I will be doing that with a brand new me. How amazing is that? I am scared and nervous. I would be standing up in front of an audience, turning around and showing my new hair, with a picture of me right before the surgery. It is a humbling thing. But in a way, it was the start of me learning to be comfortable in my own skin while all eyes were on me.

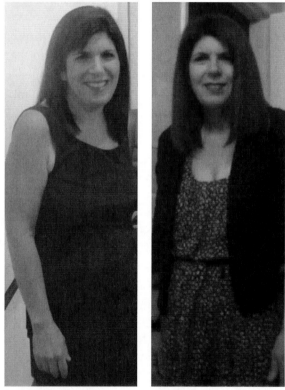

Two different modeling sessions, this was so much fun!

Gastric Bypass support group was awesome tonight. Believe or not I have been selected for a makeover to be revealed at my next support group meeting. It will be done in two sessions. I guess I will need to be adventurous and willing to try anything. Pictures to follow.

FB Status 9:20 p.m. June 23, 2011

Today is the day for my transformation, just a tad bit nervous and a tad bit excited.

FB Status 9:43 a.m. July 5, 2011

Let me be real, I was scared to death. What if I looked ridiculous with the changes they wanted to make? I wanted to be open to the possibility of looking great. However, a part of me wanted to limit what they could do to me.

Well, I met Charisse, the hairdresser and what a wonderful woman she is. She has one of those cancer survival stories that she shared with me as I was going through this process. As she made me feel comfortable, I began to open up to the possibilities that I can trust her craftsmanship enough for her to do what she thinks would look good on me. So I told her to do what she wanted to do. She wanted to do my highlights in red. Geeze, not red! That was the last color I wanted. I was afraid that I would look like my mother and I would see her face staring at me in the mirror, which is a little freaky because she passed over four years ago. Nevertheless, I let her do it.

First hair color done. Haircut. Time for some highlights. The process is going well.

FB Status 3:05 p.m. July 5, 2011

It's official, I am an MFT Intern with a real job. I will even have several offices. Yeah!

FB Status 2:20 p.m. July 6, 2011

Oh yeah......tonight I am a hair model......seriously I think the world has officially come to an end. What a year this has been.

FB Status 2:39 p.m. July 6, 2011

I don't know who is paying attention to these posts but I got another good one for whoever is listening. I became a therapist with a job today and as of fifteen minutes ago I have two office locations. Yes, two offices. God is doing amazing things. I am absolutely speechless. My new boss expects me to have many clients soon.

FB Status 3:16 p.m. July 6, 2011

I know it may seem that this has nothing to do with gastric bypass surgery, but I have to beg to differ. I wouldn't have this job if it weren't for the surgery. I wouldn't have had the energy to work and to focus my attention on helping others. I wouldn't even have taken the time to search for a job because that would have required too much energy as well. So I definitely owe this opportunity and job to the team that helped make me a new woman. I thank the doctor and his wonderful staff.

Journal Entry #63:
July 14, 2011. Today, I begin orientation. How did I get here? It seems like yesterday that I couldn't even get out of bed to complete an errand without sleeping for a long time before and falling asleep afterward, due to my sleep apnea. Now I can plan to be gone from eight in the morning until 8:30 at night. Driving to Orange County and then to San Bernardino to complete my orientation and then modeling my hair. What a different life this is these days. The funny part of the whole thing is when the nurse introduced me she asked me how did it feel to be described as small. I just laughed. Every time someone describes me that way, that's all I can do. It still doesn't resonate in my soul that the person she is talking about is me.

Seriously, how did I get here? It wasn't because I wanted to look "hot". Okay, maybe just a little bit. I just wanted a life; a life that wasn't lying in my bed. I wanted to be a better mom to my children and to feel that I would live to raise them in the way that they deserved. Instead, there is so much more.

Journal Entry #64:
July 25, 2011. My husband came to the meeting where I was doing hair modeling at the seminar. I have been scared to let him really see pictures of me overweight. I think the fear is that he will make some negative comment about what I used to look like. Even though I don't look like that anymore, it still hurts. He seemed very encouraging for all the changes in people. However, the next day when we were talking, he told me that he really didn't realize how big I had been. He said that I was right, he wasn't sure if we would have dated if me had met me when I was that size. I told him he wouldn't have seen me. Fat people are invisible. At least that is what I felt like when I was overweight. My friends saw me and loved me, but new people really didn't see me. They often didn't look me in my face. It could have partially been because I thought so little of myself that I didn't look them in the face. It's hard to say. Now that he has seen me overweight, I still don't want him to see my other overweight pictures. I guess that this is just a process.

Hair modeling has been such a great experience for me. Just the thought of someone calling me a model is ridiculous. I mean how can that adjective (or is it a noun) be used to describe anything that I do? Plus it reveals self-esteem issues still ruminating underneath. After Charisse did my hair, I realized that my personality changed once again. It, again, took me out of my shell in a new way. The other interesting dynamic has been with the six other models. We are all different sizes. When you see our before pictures, it is pretty surprising to see the changes in a person. Not just the outer appearance by far, but the things that they are able to do in life now, and how outgoing they are. How many risks are they willing to take? It's like they don't want to let life shove them down again. There is a new boldness that the fat covered up before. Also having someone spoil you in the way that the hairdressers have done with us is new and different. Many of us nurtured others but others didn't nurture us. So here we are in a place where we are just going to receive the gift. A part of me wanted to shove it away, but I made a choice to enjoy every second of it. Right now, I have modeled twice and there is still one more hair salon appointment and one more meeting to model for on Thursday, July 28, at the Gastric Bypass meeting. I can't wait.

It's July 26th, about 14 months since my surgery. I can eat slightly larger quantities of food than I could initially. I gain on and off about six pounds. I meet people at some of the meetings that I attend that are testing the boundaries of what they can eat. Bigger amounts, lots of sugar and those people stopped losing weight. Some want to know how big of sandwiches they can eat. Other people eat mini-Snicker bars and regular ice cream, which may or may not cause them to dump. They eat baked potatoes, bread, rolls and crackers and think nothing of it because they eat smaller portions. Keep in mind this surgery is a huge deal. You want it to work, not to figure out how you can cheat the system. Stay on track and care about yourself and your body. I believe in you. You can accomplish whatever your goals are. Hang in there.

"I now see how owning our story and loving ourselves through that process is the bravest thing that we will ever do."
— **Brené Brown**

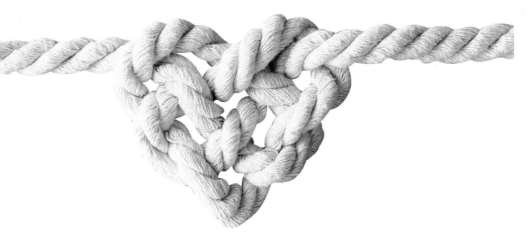

CHAPTER TEN

What Not to Do After Bariatric Surgery

Based on my own personal experience.

The following list may look different for you.

1. Don't take yourself off of your medication when you leave the hospital without doctor's prior written orders.

This is not one of the smartest things that I have ever done. Why do I constantly think that I know more than a doctor knows? Is it that I am so stubborn that I have to do things my way? Or is it both? I know for me, all I could think about before my surgery was when I was going to get off my medication. I hate taking medication; just ask anyone who knows me. I almost have to be dying before I follow through with the doctor's orders about medication. I hate the way it feels when it is going down my throat, especially now since my surgery it seems that things get clogged easier. I hate it when I get acid reflux because I swallowed the pill the wrong way. I hate that I need medication. I want to believe that I don't need them and thus, better than others. Obviously, that isn't true. It's one of those underlying feelings that is subconscious, I think. I forget to take them. I don't like that I have to pay for medication. I don't like that I have to take time off in a busy day to remember to take medication. The medication makes me feel sick to my stomach at times. I guess what I am saying is that a part of me knew that I intended on getting off all medication long before a doctor recommended me to. If I didn't have to take my medication in the hospital, I wouldn't have. But then it was doctor's orders at that time and thus I am a fairly obedient person when told what to do, so I obediently took the pills then. The minute I got out of the hospital, I quit everything, my c-pap machine for sleep apnea, everything. I was on quite a few medications at that time. What I should have done was step down on my medications according to my doctor's orders, had he/she recommended that. I needed to have patience. You would think that someone with a master's degree in Marriage and Family therapy would have some of that. Not so much. I just wanted to do what I dreamed about doing since the moment I realized that I was going to have the surgery. Anyway, as described earlier in this book, taking myself off of one of the medications abruptly caused me to dive into a feeling of "being crazy". I literally felt crazy. I wasn't eating to hide from any feelings and thus I couldn't hide from the fact that I felt so out of control. I was very irritable and unhappy. Anyway the bottom line here is, make sure that you follow your doctor's orders in this regard.

2. *Don't eat a deviled egg or anything else that could possibly cause irritation in the first week after your surgery.*

In the beginning after my surgery, I wasn't really hungry. I was only eating minimally. The second week after my surgery, I was trying to think of ways to eat protein. My daughter was reading the post-surgery guidelines when I asked if she could make me a deviled egg, which sounded soft and easy to take. What was I thinking? Do you know what is in a deviled egg? For one thing, mustard. I was so not ready for that in my stomach. Anyway I ate a little bit and wanted to die. I didn't dump, however I wished that I had. I think I would have felt better sooner. I didn't throw up and never have since my surgery. I think that would have also been an easier fate to handle. So instead, I suffered until it passed. OMG don't do this! Give your stomach some time in which to be able to handle spicy foods.

3. Don't forget to read everything that the doctor gives you before and after your surgery.

I am going to reveal something about myself that is in a way arrogant and not well informed. School has always come easy for me. I didn't struggle through the reading materials. The truth is that I get bored when I read and I find that I don't retain the material unless I can put it into application. Now, I was nearly a straight A student even when I did this. So I have talked myself into believing that I don't need to read things like other people do. Well, I am wrong. I really needed to read everything in the doctor's packet for patients before surgery, after my surgery, and every chance that I had in-between. Being educated in regards to your surgery is so important. Well, I didn't read before the surgery and I didn't read after the surgery. So, I started making mistakes in my treatment. I realized that I needed to read everything thoroughly to know what to do. Maybe part of the reason that I didn't read about it was that I wanted to be normal quicker than my body was capable of. However, I couldn't think clearly, wasn't eating or taking care of myself, and then to retain the treatment information was nearly impossible. I read things many, many times and it doesn't always stick in my mind. It would have served me better to read the information many times so that I could retain what I needed to know. I suggest you do the same.

4. Don't pretend everything is normal when the s*** hits the fan, i.e. Oak Glen when I collapsed.

I had my wonderful friends visiting at my house several times that summer right after my surgery. They came at about six weeks post-op, which I figured gave me plenty of time to recover from the surgery and be about my business. Wrong!!! I was in the thick of trying to figure out how to eat and how to drink. I was dehydrated. I really struggled with drinking water. I was also irritable and tired. Of course at that point, I didn't realize that by the end of their second visit that summer that I would end up at the emergency room once and in the hospital for nearly three days a few days later. At one point, I wanted to take them to visit Oak Glen, a lovely area with apple trees and pumpkin patches not far from where I live. I do remember going into this store to buy some fresh apple cider. I went to the counter and someone asked me if I was okay. I so wasn't. I said no and immediately walked out of the store and sat down. I was barely able to function (I now know that it was due to the hypokalemia (low potassium) that I had developed. Thank God, my wonderful friend was able to drive us home and help me until I was able to function again. Just so you know, hypokalemia (low potassium), causes many symptoms; including horrible cramps. Quite often, it would feel like my hands and feet had fallen asleep and they would cramp in contorted positions. It was painful and something I never want to go through again. To this day, when I feel anything similar, I get a little scared. I pay attention to be sure that I am not decompensating once again.

5. *Don't skip taking your vitamins. I learned somewhere along the line only 40% of bariatric patients take their vitamins. Do you want to be among that 40%?*

I admit that I struggle with following through with medication, vitamins included. I hate swallowing things. However, our bodies don't retain nutrients in the same way that "normal people's" bodies do. If we don't take vitamins, this can affect in a myriad of ways. Don't be stupid!

6. *Don't skip exercising. There is a window in which to lose weight after your surgery. If you miss it, it will be much harder to lose weight later on.*[22]

You may have considered at this point that this list is a compilation of some of the "stupid things" I have done since my surgery. I want it to be a life lesson to some of you. You can make new and better choices than I made. There really is a window that you have after your surgery. It is an "I can lose weight real quick window." At some point, that "losing weight real quick" window begins to shut and losing weight becomes harder. If you are in the first year, it may be hard to imagine that this is true. I think that part of that window is that your hunger hormones haven't kicked into place yet. That can take up to a year. So, consequently, you aren't hungry. Whatever the reason, take advantage of that year like it's nobody's business! Yes, you can and may still lose weight after that year. However, it will become harder and harder, until you are traditionally dieting once again just like you might have spent your whole like doing prior to your surgery.

7. If you feel like you are living in a fog, check with your doctor. Something may be wrong.

I take this rather seriously now. I shouldn't have felt the way I did. I believe now that I was dehydrated from the beginning, not too long after I came home. I couldn't get enough liquids down and for me that started a slippery slope of me functioning at less and less capacity every day. Please take this seriously for your own health.

8. Don't try taking any medication (i.e. self-medicate) by yourself without your doctor's advice.

Remember, you are losing weight. Medication dosages that you were taking before your surgery may not be the same when you take them again. For example, you could overdose and not even realize it. That's what I did when I first took myself off a medication and then decided I would start taking it again at the same dosage level that I had previously been on. What was I thinking? I now realize that I should have stepped up the dosage I was initially on, then, under my doctor's supervision, stepped down as I came off the medication. Finally, I weighed 50 pounds less pretty quickly and would have needed to adjust my dosage anyway. I don't even want to tell you what I put myself through by taking that medication. I never felt more nauseous in all my life. **DON'T DO THAT!**

9. *Don't skip support group meetings.*

Support group meetings are very important, in my never so humble opinion. There are many different types of support group meetings. There are educational support groups that teach you different subject matters (topics) each time you meet. There are process meetings, where you talk about thoughts and feelings and are able to share, as opposed to being taught. Then, there are combination meetings where they include both. Finally, there are individual and group therapy meetings, which work on specific issues. This helps you to identify how you got to the place you were at, i.e. overweight in the first place. This type of therapy may deal with childhood trauma and/or present day circumstances that affect the success of your surgery. As a therapist, I have the amazing opportunity to work with people in regard to this process. More specifically, as a Family Systems Therapist, I help you to explore your childhood and help to identify how it may be affecting your life today. However you chose to seek help, support group meetings are extremely beneficial and can be used as an added resource in your arsenal.

10. *Don't invite a friend to come to visit when surgery was six weeks previous.*

I know that many of you have friends that like to visit, that drop by at a moment's notice. My friends were from very far away. Plus, it was a well-planned trip that I was so excited about. However, I couldn't have imagined how "not ready" I was to do much of anything at that point, except self-care. I didn't imagine that not eating would make me irritable. I would just say to give yourself some space and time to see how you will be feeling after your procedure. Put yourself first, something that many of us don't do often enough.

11. *Don't eat sugar.*

This is for many reasons. First of all, you could experience the "dumping effect." It is very unpleasant and something I wouldn't recommend to anyone. Even if you are lucky enough to experience the dumping effect, sugar can really upset your stomach, i.e. gurgling, gas and discomfort. Ultimately, sugar can be one of the shortest ways to gain your weight back. So my recommendation is, **"Just don't do it!"**

12. *Don't drink Slurpees! Hello! They are carbonated beverages. While you are at it, don't drink soda water, either!*

Drinking Slurpees and sodas are other slippery slopes to gaining your weight back. Think about it. The carbonation can cause your stomach to stretch. Why would you want your stomach to stretch? I will answer that question, you don't. Be very careful what goes into your mouth. Certain things can be major contributors for your surgery not being successful. If you are going to make bad choices, why have the surgery?

13. *Watch your potassium and other levels.*

You already know that I went through a horrible experience from hypokalemia. My potassium levels were dangerously low. I could have died from a heart attack during that time. I didn't even realize how important potassium was to the general functioning of your body. However, there are other important levels to consider; blood sugar and magnesium levels are important, too. Again, I am not a doctor. So make sure you see your doctor and have your blood levels checked as often as they find necessary. This is important stuff.

14. Don't eat carbs without protein.

There are many different reasons for this. For instance, with me, my blood sugar would dive very badly with carbs. Six years out, and I still have the same problem. I have a blood glucose monitor and glucose tablets with me wherever I go – in my car, bedroom, job, purse, etc. Since we know carbohydrates can cause you to gain weight back, fill up on the protein, not on the, oh so fattening carbs. Keep this in mind when you are eating.

15. Don't drink alcohol.

Yes you heard me, be careful in this area. Alcohol consumption after your surgery can cause your blood alcohol level to be higher than the average person. In other words, you will get drunk quicker. Further, there are many calories in liquids and alcohol. Keep this in mind; don't trade one addiction for another.[26]

So there it is, these are some of the things I went through. In writing this, my hope is that you don't have to. Through trial and error, I found out what works for me. Hopefully, through trial and not so much error, you can, too.

Since we have a large list of things "not" to do, I thought it only appropriate to create a similar list of this you "can" do.

10 Do's

1. Stay hydrated.
2. Take your vitamins as suggested by your doctor.
3. Exercise.
4. Attend support group meetings.
5. Eat wisely.
6. Take your medication as prescribed.
7. Eat protein.
8. Self-care is primary.
9. Attend all your doctor appointments.
10. Make new friends from this process that support you along the way.
11. Strive for your "Magnificent Life."

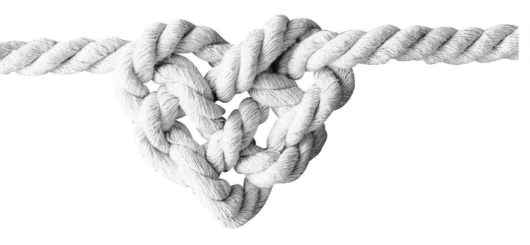

CHAPTER ELEVEN

Friends and Family

This book is for you, the bariatric patient, or anyone considering the procedure. However, I know that you have not been through this time in a bubble. There are people in your life that are affected by this choice you made. Let me take a moment and address those people personally. It's up to you to encourage them to read this chapter, as it is written specifically for them. However, you may also find it helpful to understand their thoughts and their feelings. Stay tuned for a book planned in the future, to address this very topic.

I want to take some time and address the friends and family of the person in your life that is losing weight. Yes, I am talking to you! I know you may have felt invisible because the one that is losing the weight, is often the one that gets so much of the attention. However, I know that you are going through your own process. Just as I shared that my daughter had to go through her ups and downs, I am sure you are going through your own as well.

What does it look like for you? Are you a husband or wife of someone having the surgery? Are you scared that once they lose all that weight, they will look so good that others may pursue them? I have to tell you that is a valid concern. It can be very heady losing all that weight and getting noticed for the first time in a long time. However, living in fear of them leaving you is not healthy. Remember F.E.A.R. can be an acronym for False Evidence Appearing Real. In other words, that fear could be in your head and it may not be real. But, let's say for now it isn't real because your loved one hasn't even lost the weight yet, or your loved one is clear that they are committed to you. Why not live in the present and deal with what is necessary as it happens in real time? What other concerns do you have? Do you also have a weight issue? Many times people with addictions will find another person with their own addiction. Are you beginning to wonder if you need the surgery, too? Or do you want your loved one to stay the same because you fear they will outgrow you? I have spent many years in 12-step recovery talking to family members that struggle with the adjustment of someone becoming healthier in their family system. You wouldn't think that would be an adjustment, because you might imagine wouldn't they be happy to have their loved one freed from an unhealthy place. However, change can be difficult for anyone. Both you and your loved one are experiencing this process.

Are you worried that if you don't get on the train, you will be left at the station? What is the station? Maybe it is the place where the person moves on to bigger, better things. It's natural to feel some of thee feelings. However, if you are already struggling with your own issues, then these types of problems will definitely show up as a stumbling block. Try and notice what is going on in your life and offer yourself no shame or judgment. Just notice what you are doing and how you respond to people, locations and things around you. Remember that you can never control those people, places or things, and thus you may be creating your own unhappiness by thinking that you can.

What if you are a son or daughter how does this affect you? As with my children, they were younger and their experience may be different than an adult child. Children may also find the process of change difficult, because good or bad, change is really about the unknown. Will Mommy or Daddy be the same? How will things be different? Maybe if you are a teenager you don't want to be bothered by your parent and don't even want to talk about any of this. Whatever you are experiencing, it is ok. The best thing to do is talk about it with others that you trust with your feelings. Don't hold it in. Don't use denial and try and convince yourself that you don't care. I've tried that many times and it doesn't work. Well, it may work for awhile, but eventually you have to face those thoughts and feelings you are trying to push aside. If you chose not to, there are consequences somewhere down the line. I liken this to pushing something under a rug. You push it under again and again, until eventually you trip over the rug and can't avoid it anymore. You are welcome to try pushing your feelings aside. Sooner or later, it will be beneficial to face what you are feeling.

What if you are a sister or brother to the person that is losing weight? You might be jealous. Maybe you have some left over sibling rivalry stuff and when this happens it rears its ugly head. Your family can be a source of comfort for you, and if that person is changing, you have to change along with them. It's like a pendulum that moves back and forth. If one of the pieces starts to move, they will all be moving after a while. The same is true for a family. If one of you begins to change, the rest of you will change in one way or another. It's up to you as to how that change will manifest. Will you be caring and loving or jealous and angry? One choice can be more beneficial than the other. It's all a choice. How do you want to show up in life? Would you like to be viewed as a kind person or an angry one? We all get to decide how we want others to experience us in life. Then we have the opportunity to match how we want others to see us, with how we feel inside.

Another thing that is important to discuss are boundaries. Do you know what boundaries are? That is that place where you choose to say yes or no to a request. Or, you are clear that this is something that you will allow in your life. If it is not, then you are clear that you will move on under certain circumstances. For instance, domestic violence and/or alcoholism may be areas that you are not interested in visiting. So, if your mate, sibling or child is doing these sorts of behaviors, then you may choose to limit your interactions with them. Maybe it's a way of preservation to deal with your feelings about what your loved one is doing.

Have you considered whether you are ready for your loved one to change? Or are you pondering that now as your loved one loses the weight? I don't think you can know that answer fully until you are in the process of watching the weight come off week after week.

Do you wonder if you're loved one's personality will change? If you have read my book, you know that I went through various stages of moodiness due to various factors. Letting go of the emotional support of food is difficult. I would expect some sort of change during this time. With each person, it is different. You know your loved one. Do they already struggle with irritability? What about you, do you struggle with irritability? These things show up all the more during stressful times such as this. Just ask my family, or better yet, don't. Maybe you can just take my word for this. It's embarrassing to realize that I am not always the kind person that I want to show up to be.

Try and remember not to sabotage your loved one along the way. Do you understand sabotage? It means showing them some food that they shouldn't eat and offering it to them. Saying something like it's ok to have just one little bit and it won't hurt you. You may not realize it, but you may be trying to stop them from losing the very weight that you say you want them to lose.

I do want you to know, the loved one of the person losing the weight, my heart is with you. I know that some part of you is scared of the changes, and maybe another part of you is excited for the changes. If you are the spouse, you may be looking forward to feeling more attracted to your partner, and embarrassed to tell him/her what you are feeling. I want you to have a voice, it's important that you do. You are just as important in this situation as the person that is losing the weight.

There are many coping skills for you to deal with your own feelings. You may seek out your own therapy, as your own issues come to the surface. I teach my clients that there are many different coping skills to dealing with their feelings. I use their smart phone as a resource in their life. I teach them to write a note on their smart phone for a list of coping skills. This list is helpful because when we are upset, we don't think clearly. Our brains need to calm down. However, we can think clear enough to get out our note and try one of the techniques listed.

The first thing I recommend is breathing at least four deep breaths. Why? Because our brains need oxygen in order to work most effectively. If you are going through this process with your loved one, remember to breathe so that you don't argue. The rest of the skills that I list are my own personal coping skills note are:

Smart Phone Coping Skills

- 4 deep breaths - breath2relax free app from the Veterans Administration (VA), yes this is a free app available online
- Calm app, another app that has many different free features
- Self Created Video of Calm Place, create your own video, for me that was the beach
- Muscle Relaxation tightening and loosening each muscle
- Music
- Exercise
- Distractions - TV, video, reading (or whatever works for you)
- Cooking (If that is calming for you)
- Calling a friend to help them or to vent to them (friends are a good thing)

- Spend time with a cat, dog, child, etc. (I like furry cuddly things, that are relaxing)
- Journaling (very helpful technique to write about thoughts and feelings)
- Mindfulness (Google this, there are many techniques that are helpful)
- Grounding techniques (One quick grounding technique is to list all the colors you know. It can be very relaxing, try it!)

There are many more options to try. This is just my list to help you deal with thoughts and feelings that create anxiety.

The bottom line is that you all have things that you are thinking and feeling. You may be just like the person that ate compulsively, trying to push down emotions. I ask myself, as a family member or loved one, what do you feel? Do you talk to others about your feelings? Do you feel that it is acceptable to have feelings when you are watching your loved one going through such a hard process? Only you can answer that question for yourself. My answer would be a huge YES! Allow yourself those feelings.

Where is the place for the friends and family to go and share? I would love to hear from you and help you to answer your questions and/or help you with your particular situation. Without hearing from you, I am unable to know what you are thinking. Please feel free to contact me at *www.caroladkisson.com* and share your situation with me. The more I understand, the more difference I can make to you, the family member or loved one of a bariatric patient.

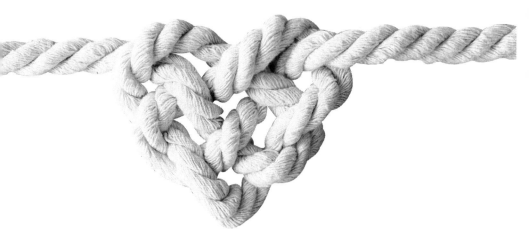

CHAPTER TWELVE

Types of Bariatric Surgery

As I am not a doctor or a medical clinician, I am quoting verbatim per the Mayo Clinic the following information. There are four common types of bariatric surgery.[27]

1. The Roux-enY gastric bypass is the surgery I had.

In Roux-en-Y gastric bypass, the surgeon creates a small pouch at the top of the stomach. The pouch is the only part of the stomach that receives food. This greatly limits the amount that you can comfortably eat and drink at one time. The small intestine is then cut a short distance below the main stomach and connected to the new pouch. Food flows directly from the pouch into this part of the intestine. The main part of the stomach, however, continues to make digestive juices. The portion of the intestine still attached to the main stomach is reattached farther down. This allows the digestive juices to flow to the small intestine. Because food now bypasses a portion of the small intestine, fewer nutrients and calories are absorbed.

2. Laparoscopic adjustable gastric banding

In the laparoscopic adjustable gastric banding procedure, a band containing an inflatable balloon is placed around the upper part of the stomach and fixed in place. This creates a small stomach pouch above the band with a very narrow opening to the rest of the stomach.

A port is then placed under the skin of the abdomen. A tube connects the port to the band. By injecting or removing fluid through the port, the balloon can be inflated or deflated to adjust the size of the band. Gastric banding restricts the amount of food that your stomach can hold, so you feel full sooner, but it doesn't reduce the absorption of calories and nutrients.

3. Sleeve gastrectomy

In a sleeve gastrectomy, part of the stomach is separated and removed from the body. The remaining section of the stomach is formed into a tube-like structure. This smaller stomach cannot hold as much food. It also produces less of the appetite-regulating hormone ghrelin, which may lessen your desire to eat. However, sleeve gastrectomy does not affect the absorption of calories and nutrients in the intestines.

4. Duodenal switch with biliopancreatic diversion

As with sleeve gastrectomy, this procedure begins with the surgeon removing a large part of the stomach. The valve that releases food to the small intestine is left, along with the first part of the small intestine, called the duodenum.

The surgeon then closes off the middle section of the intestine and attaches the last part directly to the duodenum. This is the duodenal switch.

The separated section of the intestine isn't removed from the body. Instead, it's reattached to the end of the intestine, allowing bile and pancreatic digestive juices to flow into this part of the intestine. This is the biliopancreatic diversion.

As a result of these changes, food bypasses most of the small intestine, limiting the absorption of calories and nutrients. This, together with the smaller size of the stomach, leads to weight loss.

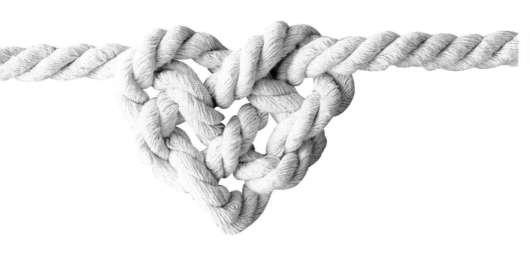

CONCLUSION

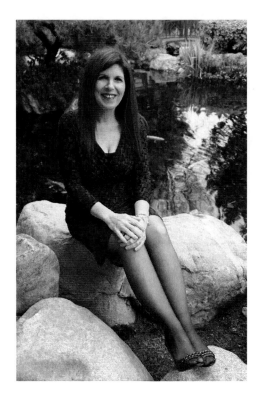

I want to say that although this story had many ups and downs, I am clear that I would do this surgery over and over again. Because of this process, I have become the person I always knew that I could be. Period. I could not navigate the path in that place I was in. That place consisted of the overweight person that had profound medical problems she couldn't overcome on her own volition. You will have to make your own decision on how you feel about this surgery many years from now. This is a personal journey for everyone and I am telling you my own personal bariatric story.

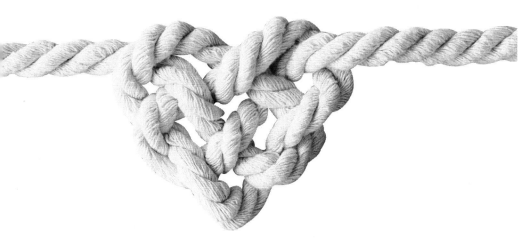

RESOURCES

12 Bariatric Surgery Resources
http://hallmarkhealth.org/bariatric-and-weight-management-program/blog/12cool-places-to-find-weight-loss-recipes-and-tips/

Obesity Action Coalition
http://www.obesityaction.org/educational-resources/resource-articles-2/weight-loss-surgery/the-post-surgery-diet-for-bariatric-patients-what-to-expect

Obesity Help
http://www.obesityhelp.com

Online Weight Loss Surgery Support
http://www.bariatric-surgery-source.com/online-weight-loss-support.html

Nutrition Resources
http://www.muschealth.org/weight-loss-surgery/nutrition/index.html

Bariatric Surgery Resources
http://www.muschealth.org/weight-loss-surgery/nutrition/index.html

Bariatric Surgery Resources – Mayo Clinic
http://www.mayoclinic.org/tests-procedures/bariatric-surgery/resources/prc-20019138

BariatricPal.com
A wonderful resource that includes forums and products specific to your bariatric needs.

Amanda Shannon MA, LMFT
Amanda.D.Shannon@gmail.com
Washington State

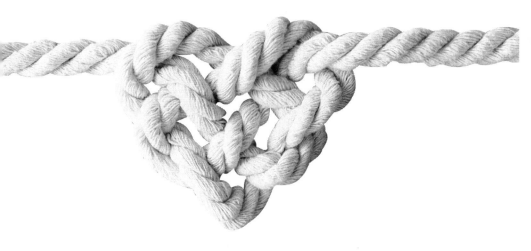

VIDEO BLOGS

Now if you see my video blogs, you are going to see someone that seriously looks real and raw. At least as I look over my videos, that is what I see. I have to say that I find talking to a camera sooooo awkward. And as I mentioned earlier in the book, I have always had issues with my teeth. I will tell you a little secret, I was born with yellow teeth. My mom said that she didn't take calcium or drink milk when she was pregnant with me and thus my teeth never looked right. I am completely embarrassed to smile because people will see how yellow my teeth are (even though I have a whitening kit from the dentist that I occasionally use on my teeth). So when I am looking at myself in my video blog, or at pictures of myself, I avoid smiling with an open mouth. So now you know my secret. Now if you ever see me speak somewhere, you will see someone very different than what you see in my blogs. I am a new person now; you might not even recognize me. It feels important for me to say, both people are me, just in different phases of my life.

As I read back through this, I also see that that inner critic in me can be harsh. These videos take courage to show to someone. They are honest, vulnerable and authentic. I hope you see them in that light. Enjoy.

You can access my videos at: www.recoveringmylife.net with this secret password— **Newlife**

Appendix A

Approval Letter

Oct. 1, 2009

Re: Referral for Bariatric Surgery

Dear Dr:

This letter is to inform you of all the things that I have tried throughout my life to lose weight. First of all, I was overweight from the time that I was ten or eleven years old. When I was twelve years old, I began my menstrual cycle. I dieted for the first time. I lost twenty or thirty pounds and it stayed off for a period of less than a year. The way that I lost weight was to eat vegetables and proteins and to frequently exercise. It worked, however, not for long.

As I got older, I began this cycle of doing the same thing over and over again. I lost anywhere from thirty to seventy pounds each time. I usually did the same diet of vegetables with proteins because I realized if I didn't eat the proteins I would stutter and have problems. Later I recognized this as hypoglycemia. The last time I lost weight was about two and a half years ago. I began having frequent migraines almost daily. I later found out this was due to sleep apnea. The nurse practitioner placed me on Topamax, at that point I was not hungry and I lost about forty pounds. As soon as the medication stopped affecting my taste buds, I gained the weight back. I also tried phentermine after the Topamax. It made no change in my weight at all. I have been told numerous times that a test revealed there was a problem with my liver. I have since found out that I have a fatty liver and that is why these tests continue to reveal a problem.

Finally, last year I was in three car accidents in a ten week period. I currently am healing from these accidents. I was not at fault for the car accidents, but I was struggling with the pain and not having the ability to get back to my life. It has now been one year since my first accident. I have painful back problems and I am healing from a frozen shoulder. As I look to all my medical problems, i.e. c-pap machine for my sleep apnea, cholesterol meds for my high cholesterol, blood pressure meds for high blood pressure, I also take n-vigil medication from the samples that my doctor received just to stay awake through the day because my c-pap isn't working effectively. My insurance company won't allow me to get my medication even though I fit the criteria. I also recently developed heartburn, which I know will get better from weight loss. I have had gestational diabetes and I currently have hypoglycemia and I know that this could develop into diabetes if I am not careful. I was also recently diagnosed with Chronic Asthmatic Bronchitis. Finally, I have very large breasts. I asked if I could get a breast reduction. I was informed that the only way that would be possible is if I am at my ideal weight. Once again, I don't meet the criteria.

Because of my car accidents I have been told that I am unable to walk or exercise in the way that I am used to and that I enjoy to lose weight. I have been directed to swim but I don't have the energy to swim because I am tired all day. I am stuck in a vicious cycle that I can't see any way out of. That is when I realized that losing the weight was my only option to have a good quality of life. I decided that I was willing and even more anxious to get some type of surgery; either lap band or gastric bypass if it is necessary to help myself.

I am requesting a referral to a doctor to possibly give me the surgery necessary for me to have a decent quality of life. I believe I meet the criteria, i.e. medical problems, sleep apnea, high cholesterol as well as a number of other medical issues. Please move this referral through quickly in the process. I am off of work at the moment and it is an ideal time for me to have a surgery like this, so that I can get a job as a Marriage Family Therapist Intern and be a good mom for my three children, two of them being special needs.

Thank you for your consideration,

Carol Murarik

Appendix B
Weight Loss Record

The following shows the running log of my weight according to my scale at home. I know that the doctor's scale and mine are not calibrated the same. I made a decision from day one to stick to one scale, so my numbers may be a bit off. The other thing that I made note of was anything else unusual that happened, i.e. dumping and why that happened. I made a few notations about my bowel movements. They were very inconsistent in the beginning. I know that this subject is not appetizing, but useful to some. From day one, my bowel movements weren't normal; not like before surgery. They were soft, squishy and messy. In the very beginning it was non-existent. I went many, many days without any bowel movements.

I know I was obsessive, yet this weight log was helpful so many times when I thought I wasn't losing weight. Then, I would go back a week or two and see I had lost five pounds during that time and everything was on the right track. I could relax. The one thing I would recommend to anyone having bariatric surgery is to keep a running list. It can get frustrating when you begin to plateau on your weight. However, if you know that you are still on a weight loss pattern, (if I am still losing approximately 10 pounds a month or five pounds a month and so on), then the frustration is much less.

I don't know about you guys but I obsess on the numbers, and through this entire process this was so helpful for me to know when I had continued to lose weight. Another thing I kept track of was my menstrual cycles. Women, you know that we go up and down in weight during the month and it is helpful to see that we are pre-menstrual so that we know why we are retaining weight or water. It amazed me in the beginning to think that I could lose weight even right before my cycle. I guess because I was losing so much in the first six months that my cycle didn't affect me as much as it did pre-surgery.

Beginning Weight 224 pounds

6/4/10   -224 surgery and lost 6 pounds right before surgery
6/13/10 - 196 lost 28 pounds
6/14/10 - 195 lost 29 pounds
6/15/10 - 194 lost 30 pounds ~menstrual cycle
6/16/10 - 193 lost 31 pounds
6/17 /10 - 192 lost 32 pounds ~dumping syndrome middle of night
6/18/10 - 191 lost 33 pounds
6/19/10 - 190 lost 34 pounds
6/20/10 - 190 still
6/21/10 - 190 still
6/22/10 - 188 lost 36 pounds
6/23/10 - 188 still
6/24/10 - 188 still
6/25/10 - 188 still
6/26/10 - 186 lost 38 pounds
6/27/10 - 186 still
6/28/10 - 185 lost 39 pounds
6/29/10 - 184 lost 40 pounds
6/30/10 - 184 still
7/1/10   - 182 lost 42 pounds
7/2/10   - 181 lost 43 pounds
7/3/10   - 180 lost 44 pounds
7/4/10   - 180 still
7/5/10   - 180 still
7/6/10   - 179 lost 45 pounds ~threw up for 1.5 hrs last night plus stomach pain
7/7/10   - 179
7/8/10   - 178 lost 46 pounds
7/9/10   - 177 lost 47 pounds
7/10/10 - 176 lost 48 pounds

7/12/10 - 175 lost 49 pounds
7/13/10 - 174 lost 50 pounds
7/14/10 - 174
7/15/10 - 174
7/16/10 - 174~bowel movement today, it had been a while
7/17/10 - 174~inconsistent menstrual cycles, affected by
surgery?
7/18/10 - 174
7/19/10 - 174
7/20/10 - 174
7/21/10 - 173
7/22/10 - 173
7/23/10 - 172
7/24/10 - 172
7/25/10 - 170
7/26/10 - 170
7/27/10 - 169
7/28/10 - 169
7/29/10 - 169
7/30/10 - 169
7/31/10 - 169
8/1/10 - 169
8/2/10 - 168
8/3/10 - 168
8/4/10 - 168
8/5/10 - 167
8/6/10 - 167
8/7/10 - 166
8/8/10 - 165
8/9/10 - 165
8/10/10 - 165
8/11/10 - 165
8/12/10 - 165
8/13/10 - 165

8/14/10 - 165
8/15/10 - 165
8/16/10 - 164
8/17/10 - 162
8/18/10 - 161
8/19/10 - 160
8/20/10 - 159.5
8/21/10 - 158
8/22/10 - 158 ~got sick, really nauseous after eating a little coleslaw at Oak Glen
8/23/10 - 155
8/24/10 - 155
8/25/10 - 155
8/26/10 - 155
8/27/10 - 155
8/30/10 - 155
8/31/10 - 155
9/1/10   - 154
9/2/10   - 153
9/20/10 - 151
9/25/10 - 150
9/28/10 - 149
10/1/10 - 149
10/2/10 - 149
10/3/10 - 149
10/4/10 - 149
10/8/10 - 148
10/12/10 - 147
10/14/10 - 146
10/15/10 - 145
10/23/10 - 144.5
10/26/10 - 143
10/27/10 - 143
10/28/10 - 143

10/29/10 - 143
10/30/10 - 143
10/31/10 - 143
11/3/10   - 142
11/5/10   - 141
11/6/10   - 140
11/7/10   - 140
11/8/10   - 140
11/9/10   - 140
11/10/10 - 139
11/11/10 - 139
11/12/10 - 139
11/13/10 - 139
11/14/10 - 139
11/15/10 - 139
11/16/10 - 139
11/17/10 - 139
11/18/10 - 139
11/19/10 - 139
11/20/10 - 139
11/21/10 - 139
11/22/10 - 139
11/23/10 - 139
11/24/10 - 139
11/25/10 - 138
11/26/10 - 138
11/27/10 - 138
11/28/10 - 138
11/29/10 - 138
11/30/10 - 138
12/1/10   - 138
12/2/10   - 138
12/3/10   - 137
12/4/10   - 136 ~6th month anniversary of surgery

12/7/10   - 135.5
12/9/10   - 135
12/26/10 - 134
1/2/11   - 133.5
1/3/11   - 133 ~reached goal of normal BMI
1/5/11   - 132
1/6/11   - 131 ~started a boot camp
1/12/11   - 130
1/13/11   - 130
1/15/11   - 129
1/27/11   - 128

From 1/27/11 to 5/29/11 my weight has fluctuated from 120-124 pounds, at least on my scale. My doctor's goal for me is 110 and on his scale I weigh more. I need to lose probably about 16 pounds still according to that goal.

2/4/11   - 127
2/9/11   - 126
2/10/11   - 125
2/12/11   - 124
2/15/11   - 123
2/16/11   - 122
3/4/11   - 120
3/21/11   - 120 ~weight loss slowing down only lost two pounds last month
6/1/11   119 ~1 year anniversary around the corner
6/2/11   118

Works Citation

Pick, Marcelle. "Barbara L., Age 74." *Women to Women.* Healthy Weight, 12 Nov. 2014. Web. 10 Dec. 2016.

Oaklander, Mandy. "How Weight Loss Changes Your Taste Buds." *Time.* Time, 6 Nov. 2014. Web. 10 Dec. 2016.

Alexander, Cynthia L., PsyD. "Depression after Bariatric Surgery: Triggers, Identification, Treatment, and Prevention." *Bariatric Times.* BT Online Editor, 9 May 2008. Web. 10 Dec. 2016.

Helderman, Derek. "Carbonated Drinks After a Gastric Bypass." *LIVESTRONG.COM.* Leaf Group, 07 Oct. 2015. Web. 10 Dec. 2016.

@betterbariatric. "It's Stuck!" *Eating After Gastric Bypass.* N.p., 26 Nov. 2013. Web. 10 Dec. 2016.

Health Guide, My Bariatric Life. "Protein Deficiency after Gastric Bypass Surgery - My Bariatric Life." *Protein Deficiency after Gastric Bypass Surgery - My Bariatric Life - Surgery - Obesity.* Remedy Health Media, LLC, 8 Feb. 2012. Web. 10 Dec. 2016.

"Body Dysmorphic Disorder (BDD)." *Anxiety and Depression Association of America, ADAA.* N.p., Sept. 2014. Web. 10 Dec. 2016.

Braverman, Jody. "Weight Loss & Starvation Mode." *LIVESTRONG.COM.* Leaf Group, 02 Dec. 2015. Web. 10 Dec. 2016.

Kessler, @nygetfit Melissa. "Got Fluids?!!? How to Stay Hydrated After Weight Loss Surgery. Slow and Steady Wins the Race!!" *Surgical Intensivists, PC.* N.p., 28 Aug. 2014. Web. 10 Dec. 2016.

"How to Break Through Any Weight-Loss Plateau-JillianMichaels.com." *JillianMichaels.com.* N.p., n.d. Web. 10 Dec. 2016.

Green, Toby. "Overcoming Critical Parents." *Bodyandsoul. com.au.* N.p., 9 Aug. 2009. Web. 10 Dec. 2016.

"30 Day Ketogenic Diet Plan." Ruled Me. Ruled.Me © Copyright 2015, All Rights Reserved. | Privacy Policy & Disclaimer, 13 Mar. 2014. Web. 12 Dec. 2016.

Albee, Robert B., Jr. "Pain after Surgery: What You Can Expect." *The Center for Endometriosis Care*. N.p., n.d. Web. 10 Dec. 2016.

Morrow, Angela. "The 5 Stages of Coping With Death." *Verywell*. Kübler-Ross, E. On Death and Dying. 1969. New York, NY: Scribner Publishers., 3 Mar. 2016. Web. 10 Dec. 2016.

Kellenberger, David, MPAS, RD, PA-C. "*Understanding Hair Loss After Bariatric Surgery*" © 2017 Kim Bariatric Institute, Accessed 3/12/2017

"Co-Dependency." *Mental Health America*. N.p., n.d. Web. 10 Dec. 2016.

Alexander, Cynthia L., PsyD. "Depression after Bariatric Surgery: Triggers, Identification, Treatment, and Prevention." *Bariatric Times*. BT Online Editor, 9 May 2008. Web. 10 Dec. 2016.

Lederer, Eleanor, MD. "Hypokalemia." *Hypokalemia: Practice Essentials, Background, Pathophysiology*. Chief Editor: Vecihi Batuman, MD, FASN, 16 Sept. 2016. Web. 10 Dec. 2016.

Sarah Jourdain "How to Improve Skin Elasticity" 20 August2009.HowStuffWorks.com.<http://health.howstuffworks.com/skin-care/problems/treating/improve-skin-elasticity.htm> 10 December 2016

Harvey, Steve, and Denene Millner. *Act Like a Lady, Think Like a Man: What Men Really Think About Love, Relationships, Intimacy, and Commitment*. New York: Amistad, 2009. Print.

Kellenberger, David, MPAS, RD, PA-C. "*Understanding Hair Loss After Bariatric Surgery*" © 2017 Kim Bariatric Institute, Accessed 3/12/2017.

Rovito, Peter F., MD. "Weight Gain After Gastric Bypass Surgery & 9 Ways to Avoid or Reverse It - Bariatric Surgery Source." *Bariatric Surgery Source.* © Copyright 2016 Bariatric Surgery Source, LLC, n.d. Web. 10 Dec. 2016.

Shellenbarger, Sue. "On the Job, Beauty Is More Than Skin-Deep." *The Wall Street Journal.* Dow Jones & Company, 27 Oct. 2011. Web. 10 Dec. 2016.

"Brown University." *Alcohol and Your Body | Health Promotion | Brown University.* © 2015 Brown University, n.d. Web. 10 Dec. 2016.

"Nutritional Deficiency and Bariatric Surgery." *Bariatric News.* T © 2016 Dendrite Clinical Systems, a.n.d. Web. 10 Dec. 2016.

Parikh, Manish, M.D., Jason M. Johnson, and Naveen Ballem, M.D. "Alcohol Use Before and After Bariatric Surgery - American Society for Metabolic and Bariatric Surgery." *American Society for Metabolic and Bariatric Surgery.* N.p., Feb. 2016. Web. 10 Dec. 2016.

Mayo Clinic Staff. "Weight Loss." The Mayo Clinic Diet: A Weight-loss Program for Life - Mayo Clinic. © 1998-2016 Mayo Foundation for Medical Education and Research. All Rights Reserved. Used in Accordance with Mayo Clinic's Privacy Policy. Advertisement, 1 Dec. 2016. Web. 12 Dec. 2016.

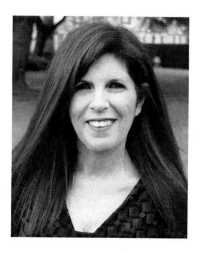

About the Author

Carol Rose Adkisson is an author, speaker, a teacher and a Licensed Marriage and Family Therapist. She currently has a thriving group practice in Fontana, California, along with her nonprofit organization entitled the Trauma and Healing Foundation. She has contributed to several published works including *When Life Happens How to Deal with the Unexpected,* 2015 *and Zoe Life Inspired a Daily Devotional,* 2015. Carol is currently in the process of writing several books that she is expecting to be published within the year. Her next book will be a companion book to *Recovering My Life* that will be an option as a packaged set in the near future. Her books encompass many topics all that have a thread of healing woven in each one. Carol loves people and feels the calling for her life has been to help people in their healing process.

Carol graduated with a bachelor's degree in Human Development and a master's degree in Marriage Family Therapy from Hope International University. She has worked as a therapist in various capacities including as a Lay Counselor for her church, as a Marriage Family Therapist intern and currently is a Licensed Therapist and Chief Executive Officer/President for the Trauma and Healing Foundation. Although Carol is happy to work with a wide variety of clients ranging from individuals to couples, she specializes in trauma, hoarding, anxiety, depression and ADHD and is trained in numerous trauma techniques including EMDR and TF-CBT.

Carol's biggest passion is her family. She is married with three children, Miranda, Brian, and Dylan. She is a food aficionado, loves trying out and cooking new foods. She has a passion for volleyball and has played most of her life.

Carol's contact information:

caroladkisson.com
email@caroladkisson.com

traumahealingfoundation.com
carol@traumahealingfoundation.com

Please don't hesitate to contact Carol. She would love to hear from you!

Made in United States
North Haven, CT
21 May 2022

19399013R00115